THE
HEALING
SPIRIT
OF
PLANTS

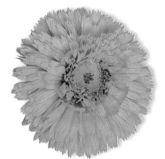

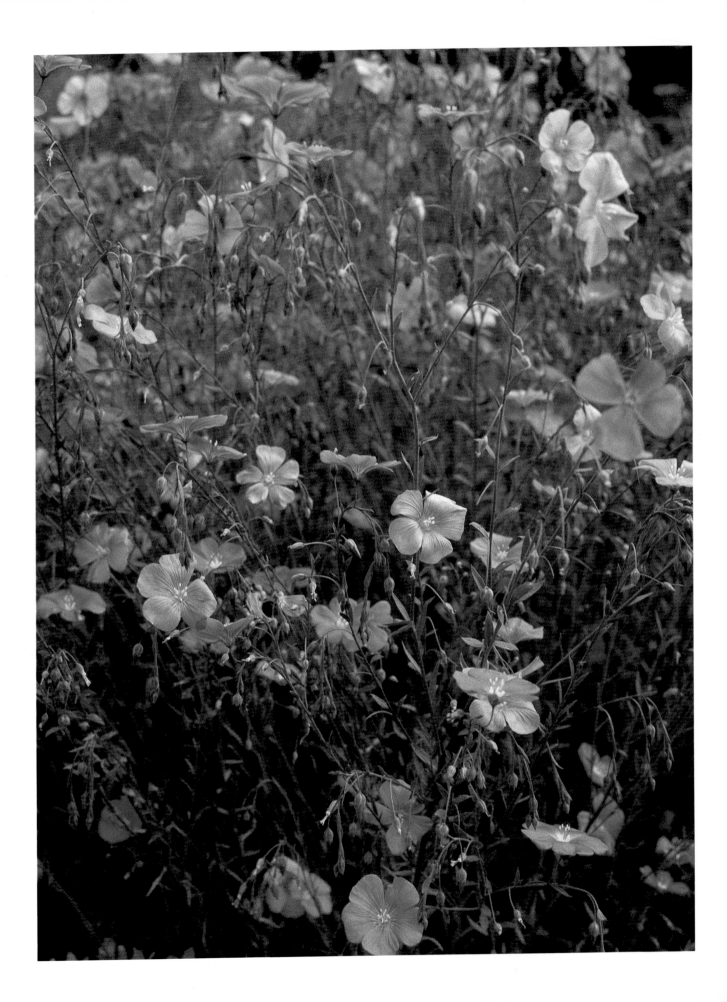

THE
HEALING
SPIRIT
OF
PLANTS

An Illustrated Guide to Plant Spirit Medicine

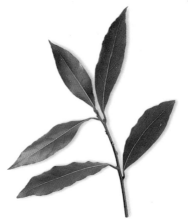

CLARE G. HARVEY AND AMANDA COCHRANE

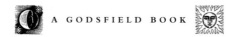

A GODSFIELD BOOK

Dedication from Clare G. Harvey

This book is dedicated to the incredibly joyous "Spirit of Plants" and
to all those who wish to touch that ethereal realm.

Dedication from Amanda Cochrane

For Jeremy and for my mother, Diana, who has been enchanted by
the flower fairies since she was a child.

Library of Congress Cataloging-in-Publication Data Available

10 9 8 7 6 5 4 3 2 1

Published in 1999 by Sterling Publishing Company, Inc.

387 Park Avenue South, New York, N.Y. 10016

Distributed in Canada by Sterling Publishing

c/o Canadian Manda Group, One Atlantic Avenue, Suite 105

Toronto, Ontario, Canada M6K 3E7

Distributed in Australia by Capricorn Link (Australia) Pty Ltd.

P.O. Box 6651, Baulkham Hills, Business Centre, NSW 2153, Australia

Printed in Hong Kong

ISBN 0-8069-7072-3

The publishers wish to thank Lucianne Lassalle for help with properties,
and the following for the use of pictures:

Australasian Bush Flower Essences; The Bridgeman Art Library p.8, 14, 75, 78 80, 83,
85, 88, 101, 107, 110, 111, 115, 123, 124, 130, 132, 134, 137, 141, 143, 149, 151, 156, 166,
176; Carol Bruce; Bruse Coleman Collection p.30, 92, 105, 116; Colour Library Images p.
39, 58, 78, 79, 88, 96, 160, 161; Garden Picture Library p. 2, 9, 17, 34, 38, 42, 44, 46, 59,
62, 77, 79, 100, 101, 104, 109, 124, 125, 130, 133, 135, 142, 147, 159, 171, 173; Garden
and Wildlife Matters p. 93, 168; Regina Hornberger; The Huchinson Library p. 10, 43, 48,
83, 87, 91, 92, 99, 107, 114, 119, 128; Helmut Maler; Mary Evans Picture Library p. 13, 21,
22, 32, 44, 51, 68, 69, 72, 73, 106, 126, 140, 156, 165; Kimball Morrison p. 122; Peter
Newark's American Pictures p. 16; NHPA p. 7, 13, 19, 22, 45, 68, 82, 84, 90, 96, 102, 123,
129, 152, 157, 160, 163, 165, 170, 174, 177; South American Pictures p. 52, 54, 62, 74, 105;
Tony Stone Images p. 7, 18, 36, 41, 61, 75, 81, 86, 93, 94, 97 113, 125, 126, 143, 148, 149,
153, 155, 157, 158, 164, 166, 172

Contents

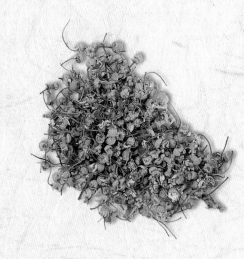

WHAT IS PLANT SPIRIT MEDICINE?

IMAGINE A MEDICINE *that has the power to evoke feelings of joy and tranquillity, to rekindle youthful vitality, bring boundless energy, and make you feel years younger. It may sound too good to be true, yet for centuries people have recognized that such a medicine does exist. It is plant spirit medicine.*

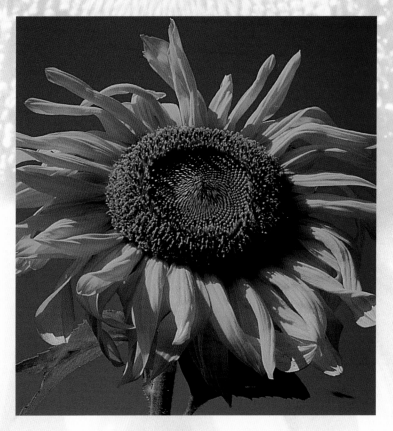

ABOVE *The healing essence of plants has been recognized in many different cultures throughout history.*

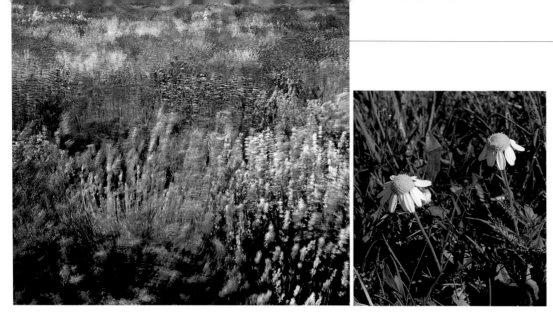

FAR LEFT *With its pungent aroma and vibrant color, lavender can relieve stress and tension.*

LEFT *The ability of camomile to calm the nerves has been appreciated since ancient times.*

All across the world and in every culture throughout history, plants have been seen as having an invisible inner essence. They have a spirit. Sit quietly near a flower or tree and you will begin to sense its energy and spirit. It may be visualized as a sparkling essence of life that endows every tree, bush, herb, and flowering plant with its own unique personality.

Plant spirit medicines embody the very essence or spirit of these plants. They are pure, natural remedies that come in many different guises. They may be scented droplets of oils from flowers and leaves, liquids infused with flower petals, homeopathic dilutions of medicinal plants, or the smoke of smoldering herbs. What makes plant spirit medicines special is their unique vibrational quality.

Whatever physical form they take, each plant spirit medicine is imbibed with this very potent form of energy, which could be visualized as infinitely tiny pinpoints of shimmering light.

SACRED BEINGS

While all plants have a spirit, there are some whose essence is of a particularly healing nature. People who have a true empathy and rapport with the natural world regard these plants as guardians or care-takers of our health and happiness because they

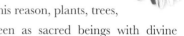

bring healing on all levels – spiritual, emotional, mental, and physical. For this reason, plants, trees, and flowers were often seen as sacred beings with divine powers. We are now just beginning to understand why.

While some sacred plants have potent medicinal properties, others affect our emotional and spiritual welfare. Flowering plants such as camomile and lavender have the power to soothe troubled minds as well as tension-riddled bodies. With their inspirational beauty, flowers such as the lotus can kindle spiritual awareness and growth, guiding us in our pursuit of enlightenment. Among the most sacred are those with visionary qualities. They owe their divine nature to an ability to elevate states of consciousness, enhance our powers of perception, and allow us to gain access to more spiritual realms.

Remedies that encapsulate the essence of these plants can light up our lives. Unlike other forms of medicine they are blessed with the unique ability to restore and preserve feelings of harmony in mind, body, and soul.

LEFT *The lotus flower is perhaps the most famous spiritual emblem in the plant world.*

Healing in a Sacred Way

H EALING WITH THE *spirits of plants and flowers has never been taken lightly. Traditionally, special ceremonies and rituals have always accompanied the use of sacred healing plants. Ceremonies and rituals serve several purposes. They not only provide a way of connecting with the plant spirits and harnessing their healing powers, they also act as a means of showing respect and giving thanks for the benefits these plants can bestow.*

Today we have forgotten this simple act of courtesy and take for granted the gifts that nature provides. How often have you sipped a herbal tea to encourage a good night's sleep or taken a homeopathic tablet to relieve a cough or cold without giving a second thought to the plant that yielded these natural remedies?

BELOW *Plant spirits and their healing properties played an important role in ancient rituals, perhaps even before their full significance was appreciated.*

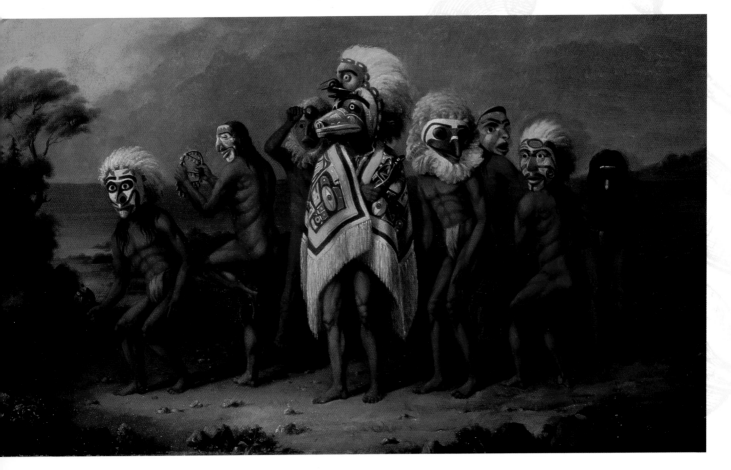

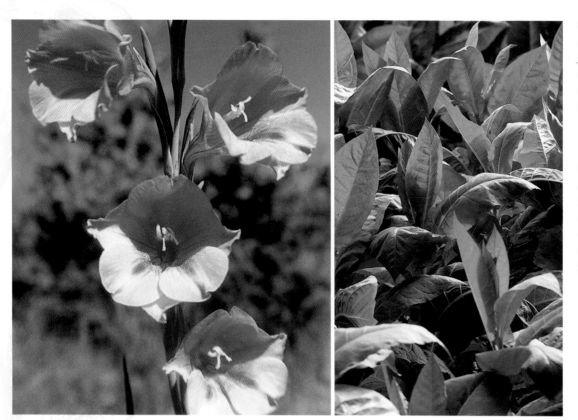

FAR LEFT
*Pink trumpet
flower strengthens
ones' purpose and
directs focus to
important goals.*

LEFT *For many
Native American tribes,
the most sacred plant
of all was tobacco. A
small amount would be
left as an offering when
picking other plants.*

WHISPERING PLANTS

There was a time when the only medicines people had access
to were the plants growing around them. Their knowledge
of the plant world lies beyond our comprehension. Ethnobotanists who study the indigenous uses of plants around the
world have also noted that different peoples seem to use plants
as medicines with amazing similarity. It is easy to understand
how people living thousands of miles away from each other
might simultaneously come to discover that a plant such as
sage had hormone-balancing and mild antiseptic properties. It is harder to explain how they come to
identify it with the same spiritual attributes –
those of purifying energies and washing
away negativity – unless they had experienced
the same sense of its spiritual nature.

People living close to the earth were so
closely connected to nature that they regarded
the plants as their friends. It is said that these
people knew the plants so well that the spirits
would whisper to them and reveal their

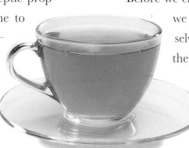

ABOVE *Herbal infusions are
one way in which we gain access to
the plants' healing properties.*

healing powers. To them, the spirit of the plant played an
essential role in healing, one that was just as potent, if not
more so, than the leaves, petals, stems, and roots. Indeed,
the Native Americans, in common with other indigenous
people, see a plant as being protected by the spirit that has
endowed it with medicinal properties. It is therefore essential to request permission from the plant's spirit to use the
plant as a medicine. Offerings are left to these spirits when
the plant is picked as a way of saying thank you.

Before we can reap the benefits of plant spirit medicines,
we need to cultivate respect for the plants themselves. Native peoples care deeply for the plants
they use as medicines, and this reverence is an
essential aspect of the whole healing
process. Before using any plant spirit
medicine it is important to be still, to
focus on the healing benefits that plants
can bring and to accept them with gratitude.
Only then can the life force of the plant start
to work its wonders.

The Web of Life

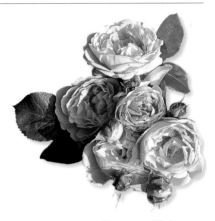

*O*NCE WE BEGIN *to see plants as living beings with unique personalities, our whole perception of reality changes. Working with plant spirit medicines brings a greater understanding of life and the role each of us has to play. Possibly the most important gift that plant spirit medicines have to offer is the ability to help us evolve in a spiritual way.*

ABOVE *Flowers can lift the mood immeasurably, especially if we learn to work with their spirit medicines.*

In all of us there is a deep desire to make some sense of our lives and to feel at ease with who we are. In our quest for inner harmony we come to realize that our own welfare is inextricably linked and interconnected to the well-being of everything else that exists in nature. We are all part of a vast web of life. At the material level, the plants provide us with food and medicine to keep us well. The trees provide shelter and cleanse the air that we breathe. But beyond what we know of as reality, there is thought to exist a more magical world, one that is pervaded with a subtle energetic force that works through all things.

Since the earliest times people have recognized the presence of spirit in this world. The very essence of human nature

BELOW *Plants are an intrinsic part of the circle of life, providing food, medicine, and spiritual pleasure.*

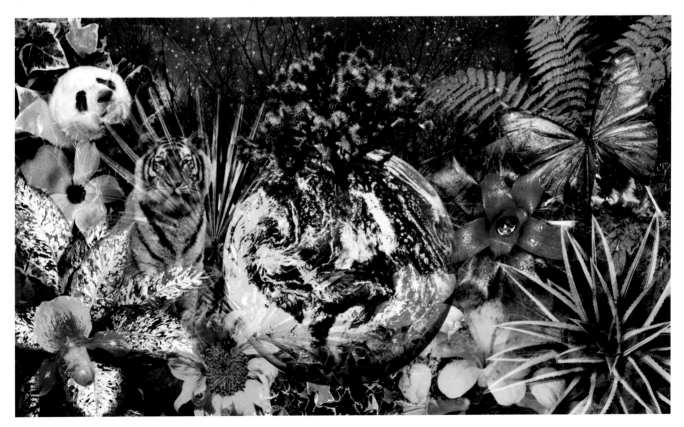

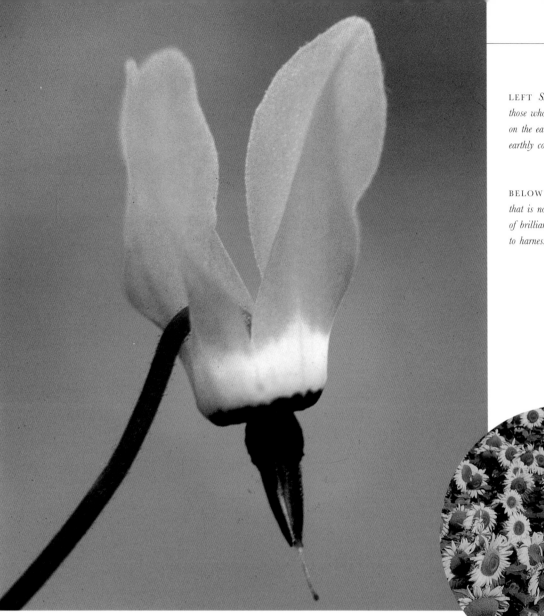

LEFT *Shooting Star aids those who do not feel at home on the earth to find their right earthly connection.*

BELOW *It is a hard heart that is not lifted by the sight of brilliant sunflowers. Learn to harness their power.*

is spirit and we have always experienced a desire to connect with the spiritual essence of all things. We are linked on every level, both physical and spiritual. It is our sacred duty to recognize and treasure these bonds.

NOURISHING THE SOUL

The new millennium ushers in an age that finds us increasingly desirous to reconnect with the more magical, spiritual world and understand its ways. This book is for those who wish to discover and harness the sacredness of the plants and flowers around them. You will come to know something of the nature of plant spirits and the various ways people have found to communicate with them. You will discover how people have interpreted the messages of the spirits and the different forms that plant spirit medicines can take.

Unlike most books that describe the therapeutic properties of plants, we aim to paint a portrait of each flower, tree, herb, and shrub so that you can come to know something of its spirit and personality. Once you have grasped the principles of plant spirit medicine, flick through the Plant Directory. Stop at those plants that you are instinctively drawn toward. These will be the ones that you have a particular affinity for and they for you. Be it the romantic rose, the strident sunflower, or protective oak, the message of its spirit is one you should listen to and take to heart. Then you will realize that the real key to happiness lies in nourishing the soul. This is the beauty of plant spirit medicine.

SPIRIT AND ENERGY

Since the earliest *times, people throughout the world have recognized the existence of spirit in nature. We sense its presence as a divine spark that sustains life. So powerful is the influence of spirit that we have persistently sought to elucidate and harness the positive energies contained within this intangible force.*

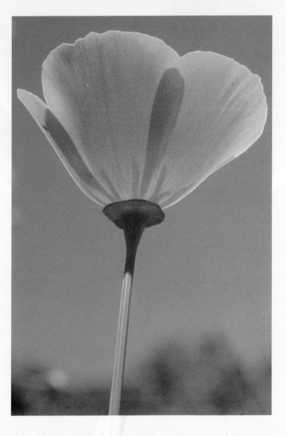

ABOVE *The fragile and delicate appearance of this California poppy belies the powerful spiritual force it contains and balances the forces of love and light.*

In the past, people from different cultures saw the spirits of the sky, seas, rivers, animals, trees, and flowering plants as divine beings. These spiritual entities often took the form of gods and goddesses whose favors they hoped to evoke with prayers and offerings.

We now know that spirit is really a form of energy. Everything in nature is composed of energy that vibrates at different speeds. Physical matter is made up of energy that vibrates so slowly that it appears to be solid. Spirit energy moves so quickly that you cannot see or touch it, yet it pervades all things. It may be visualized as a kind of shimmering and sparkling light.

Humans, other animals, and plants all have an individual essence that is made out of this spirit energy. It not only helps to shape our character but also affects our overall sense of well-being. When our spirits are high we feel energetic, dynamic, and creative. This ethereal energy is highly impressionable and our spirits can easily be dampened by those around us and our general environment. When our spirits are low we feel drained of energy, sluggish, uninspired, and lacking purpose.

Trees, shrubs, and flowers all have a spirit or essence that endows them with personality, just as people do. It is thought that each species possesses a distinct energy or life essence that can be experienced as a sensation or feeling. The impression is subtler than the more readily defined emotions of anger, grief, fear, and joy. They represent a wide spectrum of emotional shadings, each distinctly representative of a particular plant species.

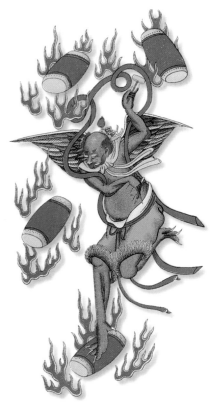

ABOVE *Spirit energy has long been recognized, personified here as Lei Kong, the Chinese Spirit of Fire.*

It may be that the reason people have always been drawn to the plant world in times of sickness is that they instinctively know that plants emit a particularly vibrant form of spirit energy. It is one that has a potent uplifting affect upon our own spirit.

The spirit energy of plants is described as having a beautiful, uplifting, and dancing quality. Sometimes this sense of a plant's essence will even materialize into a vision and the spirit will take on a form. An elfin or fairy creature may dance before your eyes, a dazzling being of shimmering light and color. Our logical, rational brain may dismiss this image as fantasy or hallucination, but all across the world people experience these magic moments of inner vision with grasses, flowers, herbs, bushes, and trees. Indeed, they actively seek to make contact with these spirits and request their help in healing.

BELOW *Many cultures, such as the Aztecs, worshipped the spirit of the sun.*

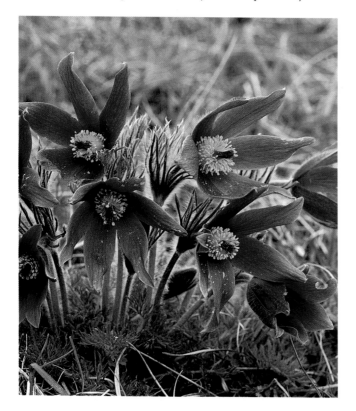

ABOVE *Each plant can be said to have its own personality. For instance, these pasque flowers have a different character from, say, billowing peony blooms.*

Healing with Spirit Energy

IT HAS ALWAYS *been a part of human nature to seek close contact with the sacred and to bring spiritual visions into the world. Throughout history, people have sought to converse with the spirits of nature, especially those of the plant world. Evidence of this communication with the spirit world can be found at some time in every culture throughout the world.*

The people of old recognized the importance of establishing a sacred relationship with plants. They listened to and worked with the spirits of trees, shrubs, and flowers. They became masters of the wilderness and came to understand how humans are woven into the web of life.

While many indigenous cultures value and use knowledge of medicines that has been passed down from generation to generation, they often attribute their most effective healing knowledge to visions and dreams of plant spirits. In ancient times it was widely accepted that plants would impart knowledge of their healing powers to those who were able to attune to the spirit world. In other words, there exists a dimension in which plants can talk to humans and we can talk to the plants. This belief still exists today. It is one of the underlying concepts of shamanism, a view of the world that once prevailed across the globe. In areas untouched by Western thinking, there are people who see nature as being alive with spirits and the universe as consisting of a complex network of energies of differing vibrations.

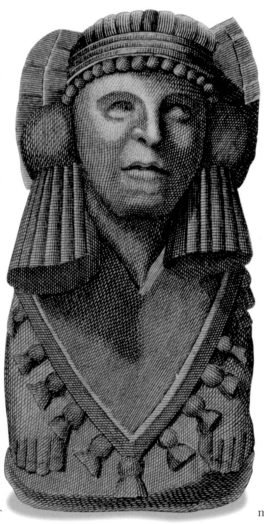

ABOVE *One of the founding beliefs of shamanism is that plants and humans can communicate.*

A WORLD OF SPIRIT AND ENERGY

The principles of shamanism are common to many indigenous cultures including the Native North and South Americans, the people of Tibet and Indonesia, the Australian Aborigines, the Laplanders of the Arctic Circle, the Altai of Siberia, and many tribes throughout Africa. Anthropologists have expressed amazement at the fact that shamanistic beliefs and practices all over the world are virtually identical among people who have had no contact with one another.

To such people the spirit world is just as real as the ordinary one. The Q'ueros are a Quechua-speaking people living in the mountains of south central Peru. They are the descendants of the Inca high priests and are the keepers of ancient mystical traditions. The Q'ueros speak of two realities: the panya and the yoqe. Panya is everything associated with the ordinary world or physical reality. Yoqe is all that belongs to the extraordinary world or the invisible reality – the enigma of the energies that are present in all beings: humans, animals, plants, and stones.

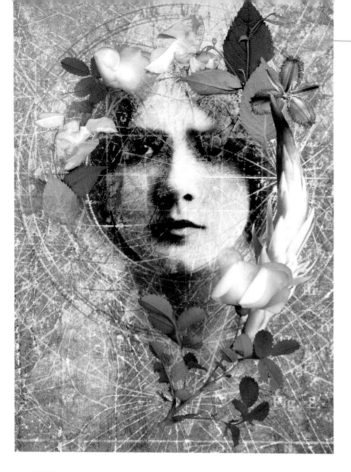

LEFT *Gifted individuals are able to perceive and communicate with plant and flower spirits.*

shamans. These people are said to travel into the spirit realm from which they bring back information and knowledge for healing people and their lives.

The ways of the medicine men or shamans are complex and still not wholly understood, but we do know their view of sickness takes into account the condition of the spirit as well as a person's emotional and physical health. It is generally felt that sickness occurs when the spirit is weakened or vulnerable. In traditional shamanism there is much talk of evil spirits. They may be nothing more sinister than negative thought forms and energies that deplete a person's life force or spiritual essence.

In West Africa one of the commonest causes of sickness is thought to be a troubled soul. Anger, remorse, worry, and the envious thoughts of others can all be responsible for illness. In the mind of the medicine man, no two illnesses are alike because they depend upon the person who is sick. To be effective the medicine must not only be good in itself, it must also please the patient's soul.

Within such communities there are certain gifted individuals who are able to perceive this world of spirits and can act as an intermediary between the different planes of being. They are the medicine men or women, the healer priests, or

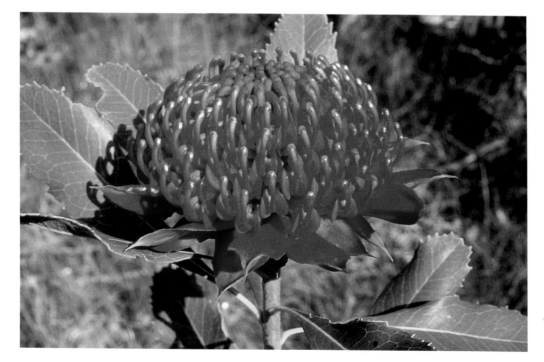

LEFT *The aboriginal name for this plant, Waratah, means "beautiful." It is the aboriginal people's most sacred flower as it symbolises their courage and spirit of survival.*

SOARING WITH THE SPIRITS

It is said that a shaman gleans his healing knowledge from the spirits of nature. Traditionally his own spirit soars into the ethereal world and there he encounters other nature spirits that "speak" and tell him which plant or plants to use for healing. A ceremony is performed with the purpose of facilitating the spirit's journey to another dimension of reality.

Often the shaman will employ drumming, chanting, or dancing to enter a trance-like state in which his spirit leaves his body. In Central and South America sacred psychedelic plants provide the impetus for the shamanic journey. At other times the spirit quest comes following periods of fasting, sensory deprivation, or meditative focusing.

RIGHT *A Native American shaman or medicine man, "The Old Bear" of the Mandan tribe.*

The Mayan shaman enters a state of lucid dreaming in which he roams the other realities, searching for ways to heal his patients. He asks for nature's cooperation to reveal any medicines and calls out to the plants for their help. He has a vision of the plant he needs and the next day will go out in nature to find it. Once identified, he will request permission to take the plant and ask how to use it as a medicine.

The healer priests or medicine men have always made a clear distinction between the body of the plant and its spirit. They say that it is the sacred properties of the plant that heal, and the medicine is merely a vehicle for the spirit. Information gleaned from the world of spirits seems to have served people well over the years. Time and time again scientific investigations have brought credence to the traditional uses of many medicinal plants.

Mingling with the spirits of nature in the manner of a shaman lies beyond the reach of most of us. However, we all possess an ability, in varying degrees, to make contact with the spirits of plants and flowers. If you wish to learn their language, it helps to know a little more about the complex world of the nature spirits.

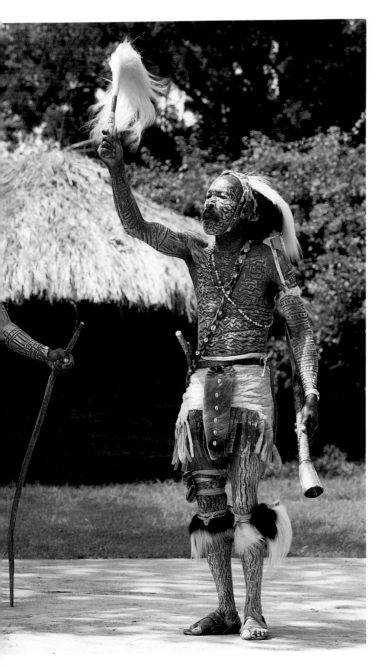

LEFT *This Kikuyu dancer connects with the spirits of nature in this ritual performance.*

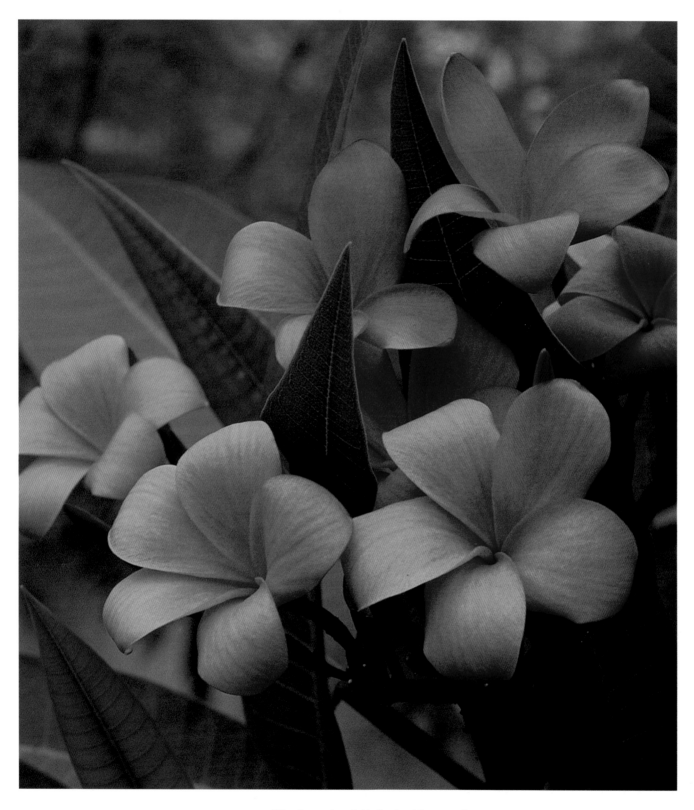

ABOVE *The vibrant colors of this frangipani flower reveal how intense the essence of plants can be.*

Spirits as Architects of Nature

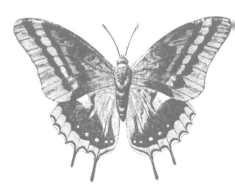

ABOVE *The remarkable life cycle that culminates in the creation of a beautiful butterfly is indicative of the powers of nature.*

S INCE THE DAWN *of time people have marveled at the beauty and order of nature. They were convinced that invisible forces were responsible for creating and organizing everything around them. Looking more closely at nature, it can be seen that complex powers are at work.*

When we look closely at the patterns on a butterfly's wing or watch the petals of a rose unfurl, it seems reasonable to imagine nature being imbued with a form of creative intelligence. The ancients referred to these esthetic forces as nature spirits. Throughout history they have been envisaged as gods and goddesses, angels and fairies. In Asia, nature spirits are known as devas, the word being Sanskrit for "shining one."

People across the globe interpret the nature spirits in different ways, yet in all cultures we find a common belief in a kind of hierarchy of divine beings or devas. Indeed many people today believe there is a whole devic kingdom that carries out the earth's natural law and keeps everything in balance.

MOTHER EARTH

In every society we find references to the all-embracing Earth Mother or goddess, a spiritual entity or energy that preserves the harmony and balance of life on the planet. The ancient Greeks regarded this organizing life force as having feminine, motherly attributes and named her Gaia, the goddess of the earth. She symbolizes abundance and fecundity, healing wisdom, and beauty. In many South American cultures people still speak of Pachamama, which means sacred Earth Mother. They see Pachamama as a nurturer and a spiritual mother who holds the secrets of the universe within her. To some people, this majestic spirit or deva takes the form of the earth angel or fairy queen who is responsible for a multitude of more diminutive nature spirits.

NATURE SPIRITS

There are the greater nature spirits that oversee mountains and lakes, smaller ones that are responsible for the woods and fields, and a multitude of others that tend to every single living tree and flower. Although these divine beings are indi-

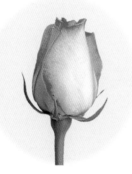

ABOVE *The supposed creative intelligence of nature can be revealed in the perfection of a rose bud.*

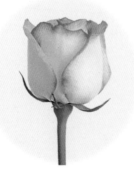

ABOVE *From a tight bud the flower develops, as it lifts its head to the sun and rain.*

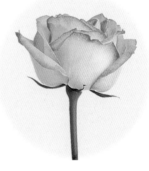

ABOVE *The full beauty of the flower is finally revealed as the bloom unfurls completely.*

vidual entities, they are all enveloped in the robes of the great mother goddess and work in close cooperation with one another.

These spirits are thought to be nature's architects for they organize energy into patterns. The energetic webs they weave are seen as the blueprints of every living thing. It is said that they work with the four elements – earth, air, fire, and water – which, in many cultures, are regarded as the components of life. In the medicine wheel ceremony of Native Americans, these elements are also associated with the north, south, east, and west points, which are symbolic of the major transitions or growth phases in life.

From a healing perspective, the presiding Earth Mother nature spirit is reputed to be a source of wisdom. Many say that this nature spirit comes to them in visions and creates an image of those plants and flowers that can help in healing.

The mythology and folklore of every society throughout history abounds with imaginary creatures such as fairies, elves, nymphs, and sprites. Could these tiny people represent our mind's way of bringing down to earth spiritual entities we cannot see or touch, although we can sense their presence?

Imagine for a moment that every plant from the majestic oak to the tiny daisy is like a person with its own personality or spiritual essence that encompasses many of its healing attributes. Many people also believe that each plant is attended by a myriad of tiny nature spirits or devas, which resemble glowing balls of shimmering and dancing light. In folklore they are represented as fairies or elves.

ABOVE *Some cultures associate the points of the compass with major changes in life.*

BELOW *The majesty of these Canadian mountains tipped with snow and reflected in the lake makes an awesome sight.*

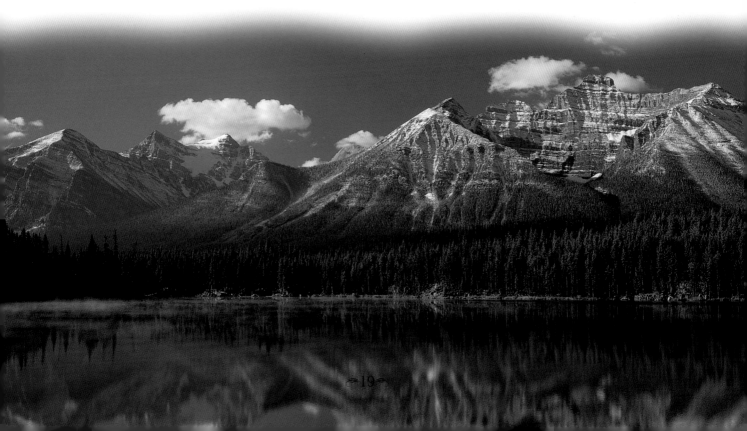

Devas and Fairies

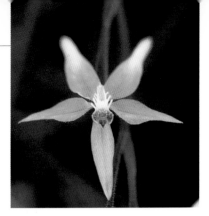

SINCE EARLY TIMES, *people have believed that trees, plants, and flowers have spirits. They saw these spirits as magical beings that appeared to them in many different guises, each form taking on its own unique energies and qualities.*

ABOVE *Delicate petals represent the wings of a fairy said to live within each flower.*

FLOWER FAIRIES

The flower fairies are some of the most delicate and beautiful members of this spirit kingdom. It is said that each fairy is responsible for teaching us how to live in harmony with nature. They busy themselves with caring for the plant. Some are thought to create the blueprint that determines the shape of the leaves, the color of its petals, and other physical features. Others assist with functions such as growth, the unfurling of flower buds, and the release of fragrance.

There is also a fairy or spirit entity within each flower. The healing energies and characteristics of a flower are imagined to be the result of the fairy's activities. Even when a flower is picked, the fairies remain active. As the flower dies, so does the primary spirit of the flower, along with some of the fairies associated with it. Some move to other flowers in the environment and assist with their growth. Others remain to assist with the breakdown of the flower, so that it can return to its natural elements.

Fairies are seen as twinkling beings with gossamerlike apparel and wings that symbolize their freedom. For while fairies are concerned with the material world, they are not bound by it. Some believe that fairies are keepers of valuable knowledge and can teach us certain lessons about life. They are said to have a childlike *joie de vie*, brimming with a sense of fun and humor. Fairies may even be mischievous and play tricks on us.

Stories of fairy folk may be the workings of our imagination, but their underlying message or purpose is clear. Their joy is infectious and their spirit inspires us with feelings of youthful zest.

According to folk belief the best time to see fairies is at dawn or dusk when the veils between the seen and unseen worlds are more transparent. To open the windows to the fairy kingdom we are told to prepare a concoction of rose water, marigold water, and magical herbs such as wild thyme. Leave the mixture to settle for three days in the sunlight then dab onto the eyes.

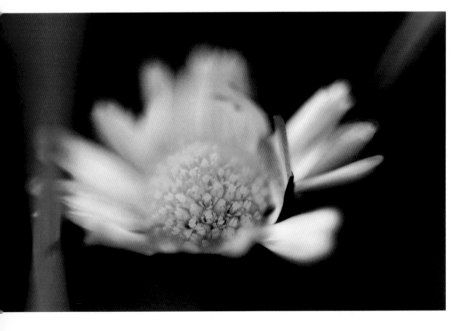

ABOVE *The flower fairy of this common, but beautiful, daisy shimmers with energy.*

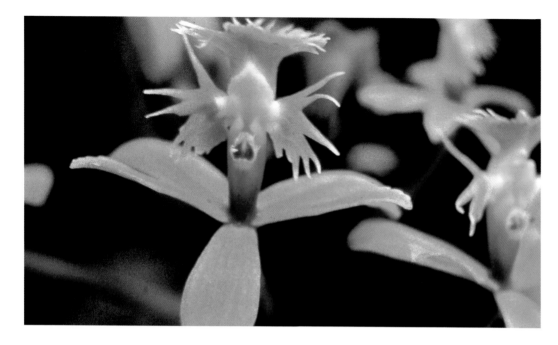

ABOVE *The angel orchid of the Amazonian jungle has a spirit that encourages us to understand and communicate with our spirit guides.*

FAIRIES IN FOLKLORE

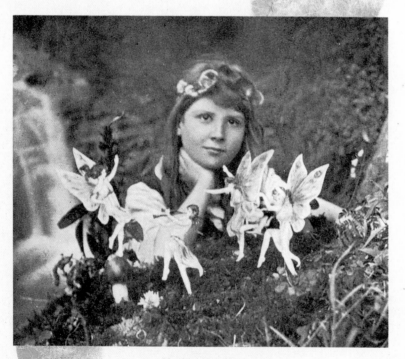

ABOVE *The Cottingley fairies. Frances Griffiths watches some of the fairies she allegedly used to play with.*

The notion of fairies, or faeries, abounds in popular folklore. The word "faerie" is derived from the Old French word *feer,* which refers to the ability these beings have to alter our perception of the world, to cast a magical spell over our vision. It is a term that encapsulates the art of enchantment.

A common English term for faerie was "elf", which comes from the Scandinavian and Teutonic traditions and languages. They belong to an ethereal realm that is known by names such as Tir na Og, Avalon, Neverland, Hesperides, Elysium, and Em Hain. Our literature abounds with tales of fairy kingdoms, and some of our most respected writers were inspired to bring them to life.

TREE SPIRITS

All around the world there are references to tree and wood-land spirits. In ancient societies trees were often regarded as the homes of divine beings or gods and were highly vener-ated. Tree worship is one of the oldest known forms of religion, and in some regions of the world, such as West Africa and South America, we may still find vestiges of this practice.

Like all plants, trees have their own spiritual essence that shapes their personality. It is possible that people living close to the earth sensed the nature of these tree spirits and asso-ciated them with godly attributes. In many cultures the majestic oak is seen as a divine being endowed with qualities of wisdom, strength, and protection. In Buddhism the sacred Bo-Tree has spiritually enlightening qualities, for beneath its sheltering branches Gautama (Buddha) found the meaning of truth. It is said that Gautama himself was incarnated as a tree spirit no less than 43 times.

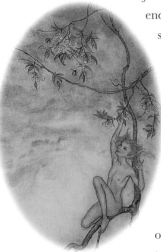

ABOVE *Sprites abound throughout literature, including Ariel in Shakespeare's* The Tempest.

In world mythology various other spirits are associated with trees. They are referred to as the jinn in Arabia, the silvani in ancient Greece, the nymphs and dryads in European folklore. These spirits are said to be so closely involved with the life of a tree that they suffer agonies when it is cut and die if it is chopped down.

Elves, pixies, and fairies are thought to dwell in branches or hollow trunks. The hawthorn, or whitethorn, is reputedly one of the best-loved trees of the fairies who gather around it and create a special healing aura. These may equate to the spirit entities associated with plants that attend to the struc-ture and growth of the leaves, roots, and so forth. Trees that blossom would also have fairies responsible for each flower.

RIGHT *This mighty hawthorn tree spreads its branches like arms, protecting the animals grazing in its shade.*

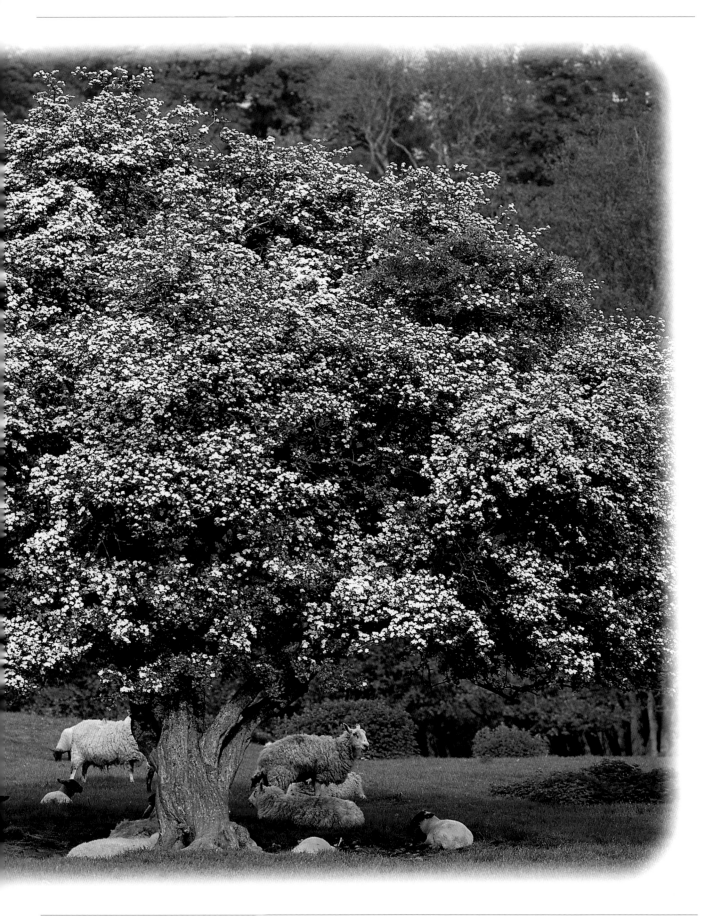

Interpreting the Message of Spirits

THROUGHOUT THE WORLD *we find plants being used for healing in many and varied ways. It is assumed that people discovered how to choose and use plants as medicines by trial and error. However, the healers of native cultures tell a different story.*

Shamans or medicine men tell how healing plants appear to them in visions and it is from the spirits that they learn how to create medicines from their flowers, leaves, bark, and roots.

Native Americans, such as the Sioux, regard the bear as the master of medicine. In dreams the tribal medicine man connects with the spirit of the bear and learns which plants can be eaten for nourishment and which ones to use for healing. Osha (*Ligisticum porteri*), one of the Sioux's primary herbal remedies, is known to them as bear medicine. Today, the wisdom of the bear seems sound. Recent research has shown that other traditional remedies such as evening prim-rose (*Oenothera biennis*) and purple cone flower (*Echinacea angustifolia*) do have scientifically proven benefits.

In the Amazonian jungle, tribal shamans regard a sacred plant called ayahuasca (*Banisteriopsis caapi*) as a professor of medicine. In special ceremonies they use a tea made from this plant to bring on visions in which the spirit of ayahuasca speaks to them of other jungle plants with healing proper-ties. It is said that ayahuasca gives precise information about where to find a plant, when to pick it, which parts to use and which are toxic, as well as how to prepare it and how much to give. Each remedy is also specially tailored to the needs of an individual patient.

Many indigenous people claim to listen to the spirits of the plants themselves to discover how to utilize their healing powers. The Mesitzo people of Peru believe that every plant species has a song that encapsulates its healing power. If you can establish a close empathy or resonance with the plant it

NATURAL INSTINCT

We observe how animals, including cats and dogs, instinctively know which plants to eat when they are sick. When we are as clearly connected to nature as animals, we are able to recognize on an energetic level which plants are needed to cure us of any complaints.

LEFT *Australian Aborigines believe the healing essence of flowers can be captured and used, an idea carried forward to the modern flower remedies in vogue today.*

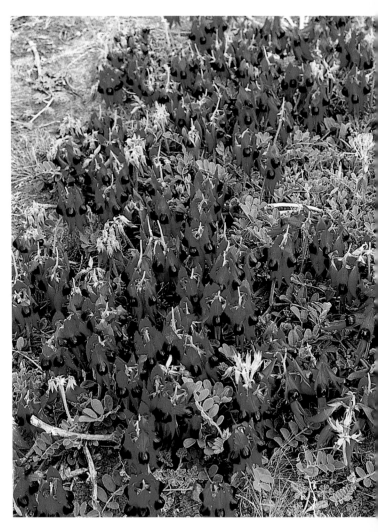

ABOVE *The Australian Sturt's desert pea is used by Aborigines for powerful healing purposes.*

may reveal its song in a vision or dream state. These healing songs are handed down from generation to generation. When sung they evoke the spirit and healing power of the plants.

Throughout history people have found ways to transform the message of the plant's spirit into practical medicines. About 10,000 years ago the Australian Aborigines discovered through their "dreamtime" (*see page 93*) how to capture the healing essence of flowers. They believed the dew drops that form on petals at dawn become imbibed with the flower's healing spirit or energy, an idea that is enjoying a revival in the form of flower remedies or essences. To the ancient Egyptians, the spirit of a plant was encapsulated in its richly scented oils. In recent years the true healing potential of these essential oils has once again come to light.

Be they flower essences, essential oils, or herbal teas, remedies that evoke the message of the plant spirit have a potent healing influence on our mind, body, and spirit. These are true plant spirit medicines.

Plant Spirit Medicines Bringing Harmony to Mind, Body, and Spirit

T HE HEALING POWER *of plant spirit medicines lies in their unique ability to evoke a sense of well-being in mind, body, and spirit. This quality springs from the natural affinity that exists between their energy and our own.*

Like all living beings, each of us is infused with an ethereal energy or life force. It pervades every part of our being and, like the air we breathe, is essential to life. For centuries healers have looked for ways to influence this subtle energy as a means of rekindling health and happiness, for the two are inextricably linked in the eternal quest for inner harmony.

Over 5,000 years ago wise men, or yogis, living in the remote Himalayan mountains spoke of a universal energy.

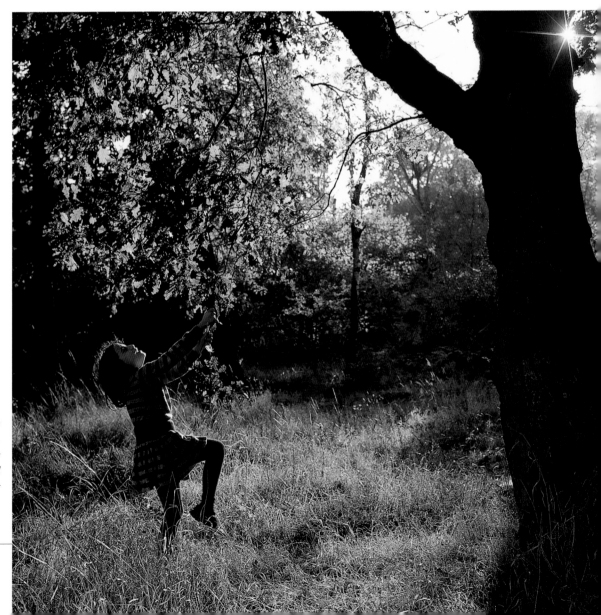

LEFT *Getting back to nature lifts the spirits, as we reaffirm the affinity between us and the energy of other living things.*

Known as prana, this energy moves through all things and brings vitality to them. The ancient Indian system of medicine known as Ayurveda highlights the importance of revitalizing and rebalancing this energy. It sees such harmony as holding the key to inner peace, emotional balance, and physical health and uses nature's gifts, especially plants and flowers, as its medicines.

The same idea is found in many indigenous healing systems, especially those of Asia and the Far East. Taoism, the Chinese philosophy that emerged during the fifth and sixth century B.C.E., sees the universe as a living organism infused and permeated with rhythmic, vibrational energy called qi, or chi. This energy flows through all things. In people, the free and abundant flow of qi life force gives rise to spiritual, emotional, and physical harmony.

The life force can be either nourished or depleted. In young children this energy is abundant and in balance, but as we proceed through life this vital energy can be disturbed for various reasons. Nowadays, feeling at odds with the life we are living and the stress this creates is one of the main causes of such disturbance. Any upsets at the energetic level manifest themselves as feelings of despondency, irritability, restlessness, and frustration. In time these negative emotions insidiously weaken our life force and leave us vulnerable to other ills. Restoring a harmonious state of qi leads to a complete form of healing.

CATALYSTS

Plants spirit medicines act as catalysts for rebalancing the body's energy. This is because each particular plant holds a special form of spirit energy that resonates with our own life force. In Indonesia, the tradition of being able to sense the energetic vibrations emitted by plants and herbs survives today. Typically healers enter a state of meditation or mindfulness to heighten their sensitivity to the spirit of plants. They also have the ability to sense sickness or disharmonious patterns within the body of the patient. This enables them to match the appropriate plant to the energetic imbalance.

Before you can begin to work with the plant spirit medicines it helps to know a little more about the various forms this energy takes.

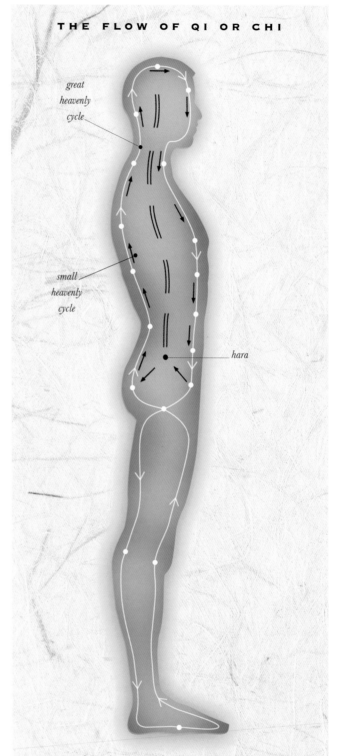

THE FLOW OF QI OR CHI

great heavenly cycle

small heavenly cycle

hara

ABOVE *Oriental concepts of an all-pervading life force permeating everything date back thousands of years. In Vedic India, it was called prana, while the Taoist Chinese know it as qi, or chi.*

The Energy Systems

W HAT FORM DOES *the life force take? The ancient Eastern and mystical traditions share a belief that the life force is not a free-floating entity but has a definite structure, taking the form of different energy systems. If we understand these different energy systems we can tap into them and work with them to preserve and restore harmony in mind, body, and spirit. By doing so we can enjoy perfect health and happiness.*

THE AURA

From ancient times artists and mystics have seen auras around living beings. Ancient Indian sculptures, Aboriginal rock paintings in Australia, and Native American totem poles all show figures surrounded by light or with lines emanating from their bodies. A group of classical Greek scholars known as the Pythagoreans made the first record of a luminous aura in 500 B.C.E. They believed its light could produce a variety of effects in humans.

Highly sensitive or psychic people claim to see auras as softly shimmering light forms that give a misty outline around people, animals, plants, and other objects. The aura is reputed to be composed of energy waves emitted by the fundamental particles of the body. Medical science now recognizes that the body does emit a weak electromagnetic field, but as yet, no one knows for sure whether the energy forms sensed by intuitive people and those detected by scientific equipment are one and the same.

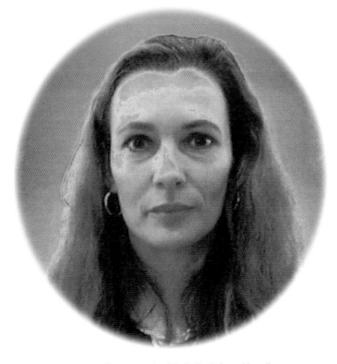

ABOVE *The aura and subtle bodies before taking vibrational essences. The pink around the brow and nose reveals a person with an open and activated third eye.*

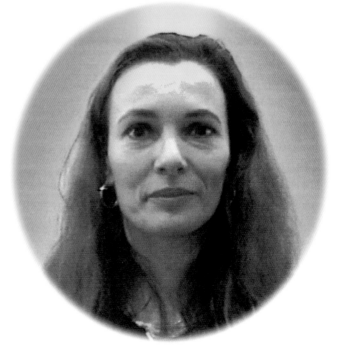

ABOVE *The column of yellow light is the effect of drawing the essence down as spiritual energy is drawn into the crown and third eye chakra.*

In people, the aura can vary greatly in size, density, and color. Its vibrancy and hue are thought to reflect the person's spiritual evolution and general well-being. Personality and emotions can also be glimpsed in the aura. Those whose auras have soft-fringed edges are susceptible to the influence of others, while a hard distinct outline may indicate a person with a defensive and hostile attitude indicative of deep insecurity. Different colors in the aura also reveal information about a person's emotional state.

ETHEREAL LINK TO THE COSMOS

The aura is responsible for our intuitive responses to people and situations. Feeling uneasy around certain people or in particular places could mean your aura is literally being rubbed up the wrong way. You may experience a shivery, pins-and-needles sensation when this happens.

In ancient times the aura was seen as our ethereal link to the cosmos. The cycles of the planets, changing seasons, the ebb and flow of tides, weather, and other environmental factors such as sunlight and sound may all be sensed through the aura. People often say they can sense when a thunderstorm or snowfall is imminent.

Imagine the aura as an invisible shield that allows us to sense other energies while offering protection from those with disruptive influences. But it is not invincible. Traumatic events, such as accidents and sudden shocks, can rupture this force field leaving us potentially vulnerable to negative energies.

Plant spirit medicines have the power to tap into the positive energy systems of the life force and restore inner harmony. The resulting upsurge of general well-being will repair any damage and give the aura a sparkling radiance.

BELOW *Totem poles such as these are an inanimate homage to the relationship between living and unseen entities.*

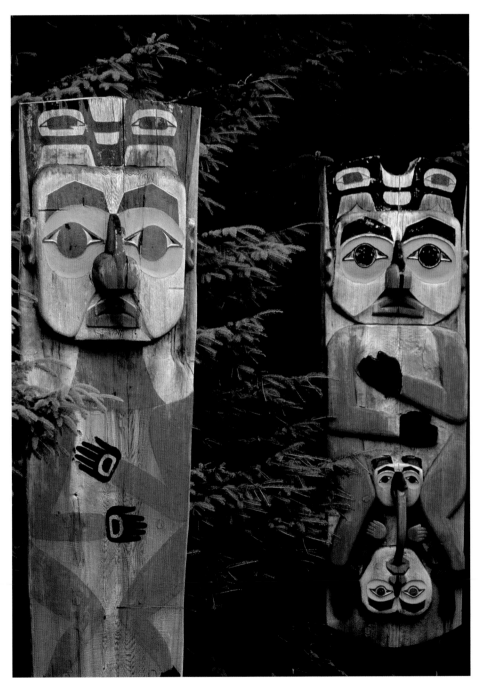

The Subtle Bodies

THE SUBTLE BODIES *are individual and distinct layers of energy surrounding the body. They can be visualized as seven well-defined bands of swirling colored light composed of energy vibrating at slightly different frequencies.*

Each of the subtle bodies has a particular function and influences various emotional, mental, and physical processes. The energy of the subtle bodies is similar in nature to the spirit energy of plants. This explains how plant spirit medicines can heal on so many different levels.

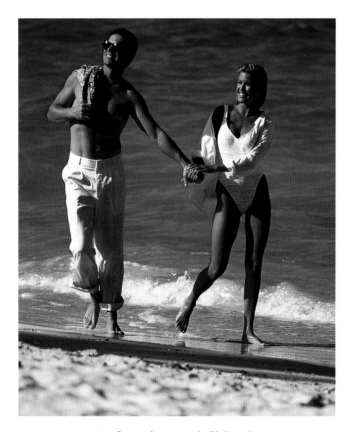

ABOVE *Layers of energy can be felt by tuning your physical presence into the forces of nature, such as those that can be experienced beside the ocean or deep in the countryside.*

ETHERIC BODY OR LINING

Blue-gray in color and linked to the base chakra. This first subtle body is an energetic replica of the physical body and contains a blueprint of all the organs. Lying between the physical and other subtle bodies, it sustains a dynamic equilibrium between them. It is connected to the earth element. Walking barefoot on the grass or along a sandy beach benefits this subtle body and the physical one it mimics.

EMOTIONAL BODY

Swirling mists of color and linked to the solar plexus and heart chakras. This subtle body is the seat of our emotions and is responsible for feelings of emotional security and balance. This body is connected to the water element. Being close to the ocean, lakes, rivers, and streams benefits this subtle body and helps to deepen our emotions and be more in touch with our feelings.

MENTAL BODY

A vibrant shade of pale yellow and linked to the second, or hara, chakra. This subtle body contains the structures of our thoughts and ideas. It enables us to think clearly and rationally. It is connected to the air element. Fresh air, especially pure, unpolluted sea and mountain air, benefits this subtle body and helps to inspire and encourage assimilation of new knowledge and to nurture wisdom.

ASTRAL BODY

Soft multicolored and linked to the solar plexus and heart chakras. It encapsulates the entire personality, facilitates an intuitive understanding of events and the flow of life. It is connected to the water element, and being close to water encourages intuition, compassion, and nurturing qualities.

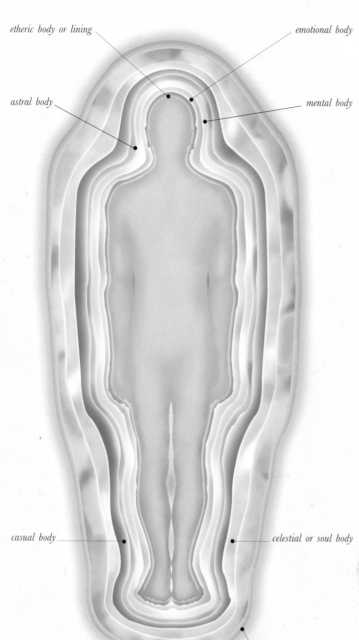

etheric body or lining

emotional body

astral body

mental body

casual body

celestial or soul body

spiritual or illuminated body

etheric envelope

CAUSAL BODY

Crystal-clear, intensely blue, and linked to the throat chakra. The seat of our willpower, it facilitates interaction with other people and events, allowing us to fulfill our personal destinies. It is the gateway to higher consciousness.

CELESTIAL OR SOUL BODY

Vibrantly luminous and golden and linked to the third eye chakra. This subtle body houses our spiritual essence and is, in a sense, the higher self that allows the soul to move freely through us.

SPIRITUAL OR ILLUMINATED BODY

A shimmering composition of pastel colors and linked to the heart chakra. It represents a fusion of the whole subtle anatomy with the physical body. Our basic energetic imprint resides within this subtle body. Connected to the fire element, this energy band benefits from natural sunlight, flickering flames from candles, and fires, which help to stimulate a high sense of spirituality, faith, and enthusiasm, awakening spiritual insight. On a physical level, warmth and light stimulate the metabolism and circulation.

ETHERIC ENVELOPE

This forms a protective outer coating around the subtle bodies.

LEFT *The seven subtle bodies each influence a particular emotional, mental, or physical process.*

The Chakras

THE WORD CHAKRA *is the ancient Sanskrit word for wheel. Indian yogis were the first to write about the seven chakras in the body. They are often depicted as vibrantly colored flowerlike structures with many petals that are attached by invisible threads to the spine.*

The chakras are believed to be power centers that draw in life force and send it coursing through our systems. They can be likened to energy transformers that receive, assimilate, and transmit various types of energy. Each chakra has its own "pulse rate" or note and vibrates at a slightly different frequency than each of the others.

The seven chakras connect with the major glands of the endocrine system and influence different aspects of our physical and psychological health. If a chakra is impaired problems can occur at these levels. Imbalance in the solar plexus chakra is linked to addictive or compulsive behavior, excessive anger or fear, sleep problems, and all kinds of psychosomatic conditions. Imbalance in the heart chakra signifies problems with personal relationships, inner conflict or turmoil, and feelings of loneliness.

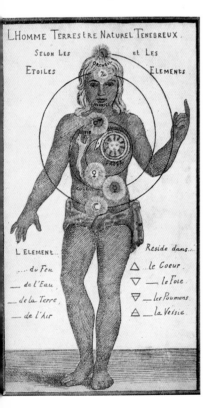

LEFT *Representation of the chakras, power centers said to connect with the body's glands.*

FIRST, OR BASE, CHAKRA
Position – situated at the base of the spine.
Function – basic raw energy.
Color – red.
Physical connections – large intestine, legs, feet, skeletal structure.
Psychological influences – connecting with the earth (grounding), survival, letting go of emotional tension.
Plants with affinity for this chakra – red clover, hawthorn.

SECOND, OR HARA, CHAKRA
Position – situated at the center of the abdomen, just below the navel.
Function – seat of power and vitality.
Color – orange.
Physical connections – ovaries, testicles, uterus, bladder, circulation.
Psychological influences – sexuality, creativity.
Plants with affinity for this chakra – jasmine, rose.

THIRD, OR SOLAR PLEXUS, CHAKRA
Position – situated above the navel.
Function – seat of the emotions.
Color – yellow.
Physical connections – adrenal glands, solar plexus, spleen, pancreas, stomach.
Psychological influences – feeling empowered and being in control.
Plants with affinity for this chakra – sage, camomile.

FOURTH, OR HEART, CHAKRA
Position – situated in the center of the chest.
Function – self-love and universal goodwill.
Color – green.
Physical connections – heart, thymus gland, immune system, circulatory system, lungs and respiratory system.
Psychological influences – understanding, compassion, unconditional love.
Plants with affinity for this chakra – passionflower, yellow ginger, hawthorn.

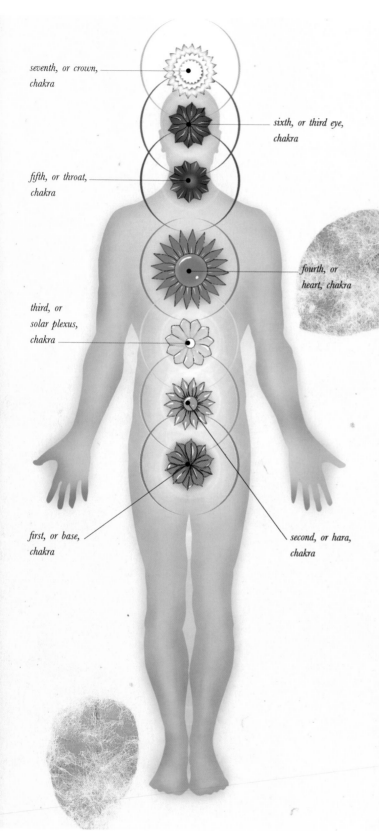

seventh, or crown, chakra

sixth, or third eye, chakra

fifth, or throat, chakra

fourth, or heart, chakra

third, or solar plexus, chakra

first, or base, chakra

second, or hara, chakra

FIFTH, OR THROAT, CHAKRA

Position – situated in the throat.

Function – center of trust.

Color – turquoise.

Physical connections – thyroid, parathyroid, lymphatic system, immune system, neurological system.

Psychological influences – trust, expression, creativity, communication.

Plants with affinity for this chakra – frangipani, basil.

SIXTH, OR THIRD EYE, CHAKRA

Position – situated in the center of the forehead.

Function — perception, discernment, clairvoyance.

Color – indigo.

Physical connections – the pituitary gland, left-brain hemisphere, central nervous system.

Psychological influences – clarity and insight, interest in spiritual issues.

Plant with affinity for this chakra – ginseng, myrrh.

SEVENTH, OR CROWN, CHAKRA

Position – situated at the crown of the head.

Function – seat of consciousness.

Color – white.

Physical connections – pineal gland, right-brain hemisphere, the ancient mammalian brain.

Psychological influences – intuition, to be open and have faith, connection to higher energies or realms.

Plants with affinity for this chakra – sandalwood, lotus.

LEFT *The chakras, often represented as flowerheads, are each associated with a color and have an affinity with particular plants.*

The Meridians

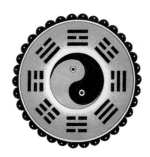

I**N TRADITIONAL** F**AR** *Eastern medicine the subtle energy or life force, referred to in Chinese as qi and in Japanese as ki, flows along a system of channels known as meridians. These channels form an intricate web through the body, like a second nervous system.*

The first reference to this energy network is found in the Nei Ching or Yellow Emperor's Classic of Internal Medicine, which is around 4,500 years old. There are 12 main meridians and each is associated with a different organ system or function. They are the heart, small intestine, bladder, kidney, gallbladder, liver, lungs, colon, stomach, and spleen, plus two organs not recognized in Western medicine – the pericardium, which controls circulation and influences sexual activity, and the triple warmer, which controls glandular activity and acts as the body's thermostat. There are a further eight energy channels known as the extraordinary meridians, which hover in between the etheric and physical bodies. Through these meridians it is possible to influence our physical vitality and improve our state of mind.

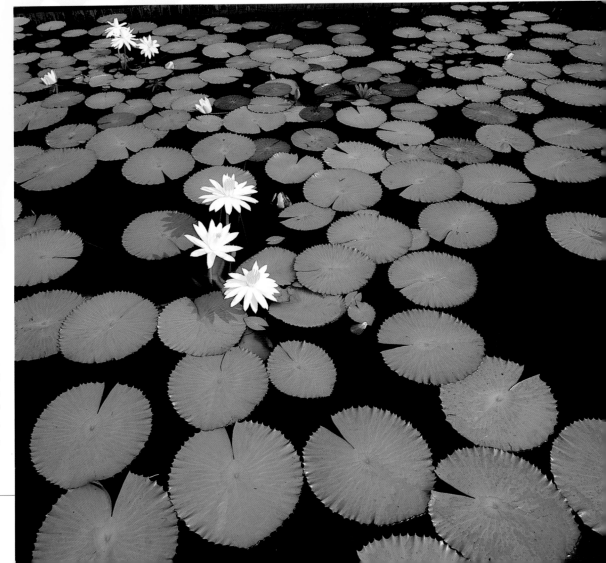

RIGHT *Far Eastern beliefs have had influence around the world. The "Lotus" water lily has symbolism in much Oriental thinking.*

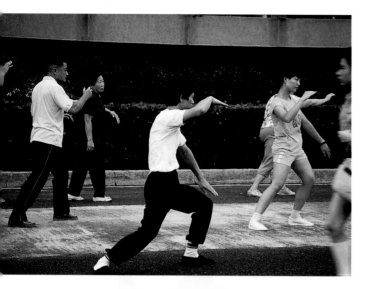

LEFT *Many Chinese people practice their T'ai Chi in public parks on their way to work, as shown here in Taipei.*

in terms of their yin and yang qualities and are used in a highly specific way to rebalance these forces and the energy flow along the meridians.

QI GONG AND T'AI CHI

Over the years Chinese physicians developed various ways to preserve this balance to maintain a sense of well-being. The flowing movement of Qi Gong and T'ai Chi use knowledge of the meridians to clear energy blockages and prevent ill-health. There are Qi Gong masters who have the ability to diagnose illness at a distance by reading the subtle anatomy. They say any illness can be explained as an energy blockage in the body. Circulation and movement of the subtle energy can clear this blockage and therefore heal the illness.

YIN AND YANG

Traditional Chinese medicine maintains that good health and peace of mind are inextricably linked to the smooth and even flow of qi through the body. It also emphasizes the importance of balancing two complementary yet opposing forces known as yin and yang. The yin force is female, passive, and tranquil. It represents dark, cold, and moist qualities. The yang force is male, aggressive, and stimulating. It represents light, heat, and dry qualities. Blockages of qi energy and imbalances in yin and yang are seen as lying at the root of physical illnesses and emotional problems as well as spiritual insecurities. In Chinese medicine, plant remedies are described

ACUPUNCTURE

Dotted along the meridians are key points – acupuncture points – that act as amplifiers and pass energy from one point to another. You could visualize them as tiny sparkling lights scattered over the body. They are places where it is possible to tap into the meridians and affect the energy flow through them. Techniques such as acupressure and acupuncture work to remove blockages and restore the smooth and even flow of qi.

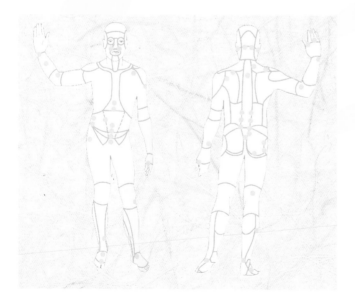

RIGHT *Age is no barrier to achievement of the physical and mental benefits of T'ai Chi.*

LEFT *The position of the meridians in the body.*

Working with the Energy Systems to Fine Tune your Sensitivity

FOR SIMPLICITY, THE *various energy systems are considered separate yet they are all interlinked and constantly interact with each other. They work together as an energetic whole that may be affected by our lifestyle and how we interact with everything around us. By learning to harmonize and attune to our subtle energies, we expand our perception in ways that allow us to sense the more ethereal forms of energy around us. Your eyes will open to a world full of wonder, joy, and charm.*

ENERGY IN HARMONY

The subtle bodies may be visualized as diaphanous layers held in place with thin membranes that separate yet allow them to diffuse into one another. They enable our spiritual essence to integrate harmoniously with our physical body and act as a kind of bridge that enables us to extend our conscious-ness from the physical world to the less tangible and more subtle and spiritual realms of reality.

All seven subtle bodies enter and leave the body through the chakras, which can be likened to energetic whirlpools. When the chakras work smoothly, energetic information passes freely through the whole subtle anatomy to preserve

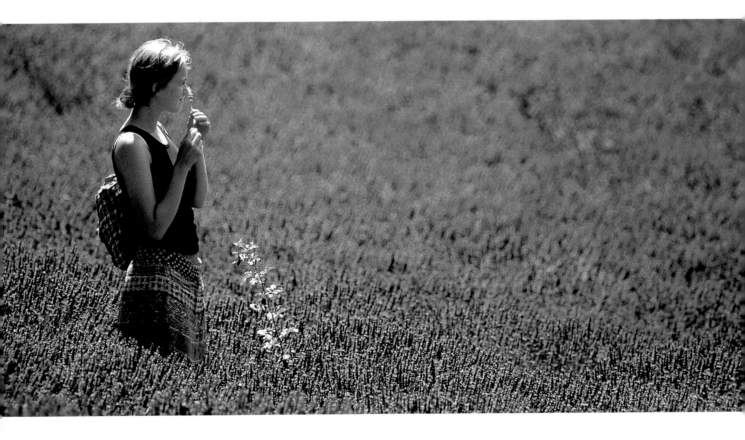

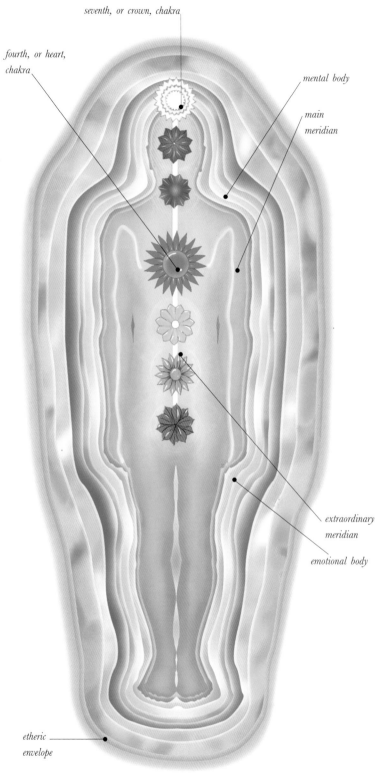

LEFT Learning to harmonize the energies within nature can improve well-being.

perfect harmony and balance. The eight extraordinary meridians, which link up with the subtle bodies and the aura, act as a sort of energy reservoir. Their prime function is to feed the main meridians with energy, qi or life force. The most important extraordinary meridian travels straight up and down the center of the body, connecting directly with the major chakras.

SUBTLE ANATOMY AND THE AURA

The aura has a special role to play because the whole subtle anatomy is infused with its energy. The stronger and more vibrant your auric field, the easier it is to sense the energies of nature. The aura reflects your inner vitality. The more balanced and healthy you are, the greater your auric field. This forcefield can radiate about 3–4ft/1–1.2m from the body but in ill-health the aura shrinks back close to the body to conserve vital energy. The aura is weakened by a poor diet, lack of fresh air, exercise, and rest as well as too much stress, tobacco, and social drugs such as coffee and alcohol. The abuse of narcotic drugs is said to create holes in the aura.

NATURE SPIRITS AS REVITALIZERS

It is said that the nature spirits play a role in building and maintaining our subtle anatomy. They influence all the energy systems, keeping the aura vibrant and clear while ensuring the smooth flow of energy if we let them.

Little wonder then that we find the remedies inspired by the spirits of plants are drawn to certain subtle bodies, chakras, meridians, or auras. Flowers and their essences have a special affinity with the subtle bodies, while the fragrant essential oils of plants are often drawn to the meridians. By revitalizing and rebalancing the subtle energies, plant spirit medicines refine and clarify your perception of other energies. As powers of insight and intuition are fine-tuned, you will become naturally drawn to the plants that will take care of you. Utilize these for their rejuvenating qualities if you feel that your aura is weak, and to maintain your general vitality and energy flow.

seventh, or crown, chakra

fourth, or heart, chakra

mental body

main meridian

extraordinary meridian

emotional body

etheric envelope

FAR LEFT The scent of lavender calms the spirit and leaves you soothed and relaxed.

ABOVE The healthier the person, the farther a force field infused with energy will be radiated as an aura.

HEALING IN A SACRED WAY

THERE IS NOTHING *mysterious* or *mystical* about healing in a sacred way. It simply stresses the importance of connecting with spirit. If we wish to harness the therapeutic powers of plants we must request permission from their flowers, leaves, or roots and give thanks for these precious gifts.

In ancient societies, this approach to healing was commonplace and still exists amongst people who follow the old traditions. As caretakers of our physical, emotional, and spiritual well-being, healing plants are treated with reverence and respect.

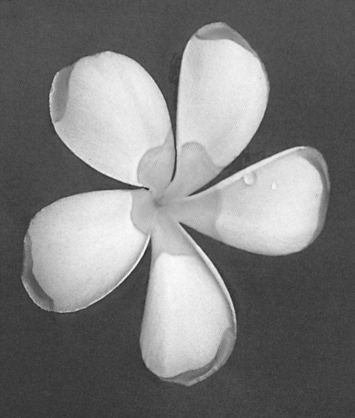

SACRED BEGINNINGS

The first step toward sacred healing lies in establishing close relationships with the plants themselves. How often have you walked in the woods or spent time in your garden without really paying attention to the flowers, trees, and shrubs growing there? You may be delighted when your favorite rose has burst into bloom, but do you ever sit with it for a while and observe it closely, admiring the velvety texture and translucent appearance of its petals?

In our urban existence, we have become increasingly detached from nature and have lost a kind of knowledge that belongs to those living close to the earth. In Columbia, the Barasana Indians can identify all their tree species without having to refer to their fruits or flowers, something that would defy even the most knowledgeable botanist. In most shamanic cultures, people not only recognize but come to know their plants intimately. They develop relationships with plants akin to those we establish with other people.

Before using any plant for healing, it is respectful to ask its permission. To take without asking is considered an insult by most native peoples. To the Native Americans, offering prayers and tobacco helps to establish sacred relationships with plants.

Ceremonies play an important role in sacred healing. No matter how bizarre they may appear to outsiders, the ceremonies are simply a way of setting the scene. They evoke a sacred atmosphere that facilitates contact with the spirits of plants and creates conditions that are conducive to healing.

If we wish to work with the spirits of plants we must first find our own peace of mind. Simple meditative techniques and ceremonies can be practiced by anyone and offer a means of evoking inner stillness.

Turning inward to look at our inner selves and examine our more spiritual sides is not the same as switching off. It actually enhances our perceptive powers so that we can see and hear things that we simply do not notice as we go about our frenetic daily lives.

ABOVE Learn how to meditate to calm yourself and look deep inside for spiritual peace.

Connecting with Plant Spirits

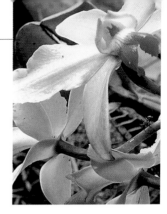

W E CAN ALL *sense the spirits or devas of plants. To hear their silent messages is a natural gift belonging to everyone, not just a selected few. But it is an art that needs cultivating by opening yourself up to the beauty of the natural world.*

ABOVE *The tropical beauty of an orchid is a favorite for many people but too lavish for others.*

When you first try to connect with the spirit of a plant, you may experience its presence as a vague feeling or sensation, nothing very tangible, and you mustn't try too hard. You must also be realistic; you are unlikely at first to see fairies appearing to you and actually dancing before your eyes. But with patience and perseverance the veil of reality will lift momentarily to reveal the plant's true nature, and its spiritual and ethereal plane will become clear.

RETURN TO NATURE

To begin with try to spend as much time in the presence of trees, plants, and flowers as possible. To establish a sacred relationship with plants you need to understand, respect, and care for them. Notice how and where they grow, the shape of their leaves, the color and texture of their flowers, the changes that occur with the seasons. What impression does a tree or flower make on you? How does it feel when you

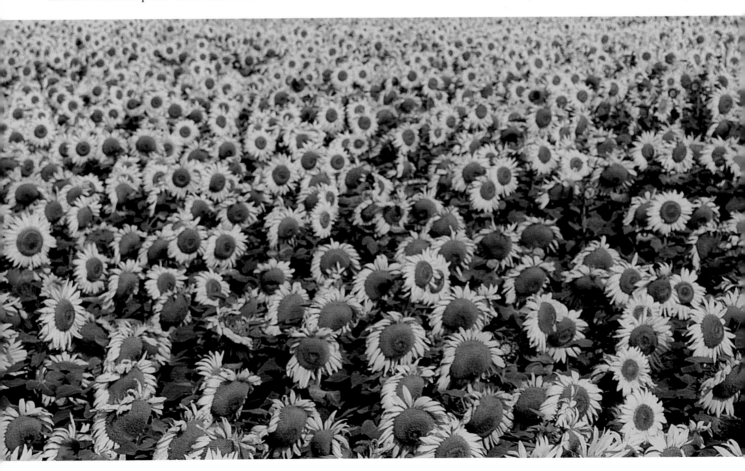

pick the plant? These are the first steps toward making deeper contact with the plant's spirit.

ATTUNING TO THE PLANT SPIRITS OR DEVAS

Have you ever gazed into someone's eyes and seen their soul? The same thing can happen with plants such as trees and flowers. To connect or attune to the spirit of a plant, begin with your favorite flower.

Find a time when you are not likely to be disturbed and sit quietly holding the flower in your cupped hands. Your mind should be clear so that thoughts can come and go freely. Consider its appearance, color, feel, scent, and general demeanor. Is it, for example, open and joyous like a sunflower or shy and demure like a bluebell? Make a note of any feelings or emotions that well up inside you.

Relax, close your eyes, and feel the flower filling your whole being. Hold the image of the flower inside your head. You may see a shimmering ball of soft color that seems to dance above the petals. Do this over and over again. With time you may find that the shimmering ball takes the shape of a tiny gossamer being, but don't expect miracles. It may whisper to you in a magical tinkling voice, sharing its purpose and the purpose of its flower.

Repeat the exercise with other flowers you are drawn toward. It helps to sit among the flowers, for instance, in a field of poppies, cornflowers, or sunflowers, on a carpet of bluebells, or in a garden of roses.

Next, go to a place of natural beauty and sit quietly for a while by a plant or tree that catches your eye. Follow the same technique as you used for attuning to the flowers. It may help to take a notebook along with you and jot down your impressions. Feel satisfied with what you receive. Some people may see faces in shrubs or flowers, but others never do. Whatever you experience, you will certainly sense the presence of the spirits.

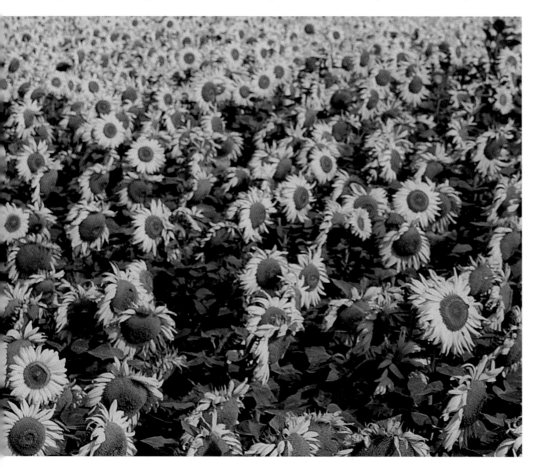

LEFT *Each flower can produce a different emotional response. By discovering the ways in which individual plants affect your mood, you help yourself to be uplifted, calmed, cheered, soothed – whatever you need. Sitting in a field of sunflowers has an extraordinary uplifting effect.*

BELOW *Sit in quiet contemplation among the trees and feel their presence.*

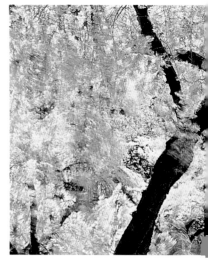

*Eyes can see
inner reality*

*Powers of perception
are awakened*

LEFT *It is not difficult
to meditate, and the
benefits are enormous.*

TECHNIQUES FOR MEDITATION

Inner stillness can open your eyes to another reality. Closing the eyes and withdrawing from the outside world is the most effective means of awakening and heightening our underused powers of perception.

To the ancients, the process of going within themselves by meditating was seen as a vital way of connecting with all that is divine and spiritual. Simple forms of meditation enable us to enter the realm of our dreams and in doing so become increasingly sensitive to the spirits and energies around us.

Throughout history, people have discovered and developed various ways to rise above the mundane reality. In many cultures, people regarded certain plants with mind-expanding

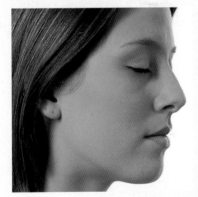
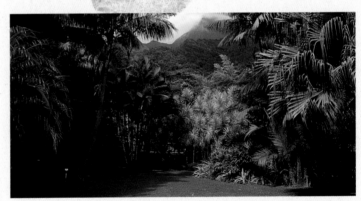

NATURE VISUALIZATION

This is a kind of day-dreaming that allows your mind to wander wherever it chooses. Find a place to sit comfortably and close your eyes, then mentally transport yourself to a place in nature where you feel most at home. It may be in the mountains, in a beautiful garden, or by the ocean. You might, for example, visualize yourself strolling along a cliff path looking out across the azure ocean. Once you are there try to sense the sun's warmth on your skin, feel a light ocean breeze playing in your hair, and hear the gentle roar of the waves. Breathe in the fresh sea air and watch the way light shimmers on the water's surface. Sink deeper and deeper into stillness. Stay there for between 15 and 20 minutes then slowly open your eyes and gently return to reality.

qualities as sacred because they enhance levels of perception and bring spiritual insights.

In Indonesia, the Menangkabau medicine men seek sacred visions by traveling deep into the jungle or to the top of high mountains where they await visitations from the spirits. In China, the Taoist priests relied on processes such as visualization and breath control to alter states of consciousness.

TWO SIMPLE TECHNIQUES

Here are two simple meditation techniques to enhance your perception of the natural world while evoking feelings of bliss and inner tranquillity.

*Insights can
be spiritual*

*Slow breathing
induces calm*

RIGHT *With practice,
you can learn to enjoy
a little piece of calm
wherever you are.*

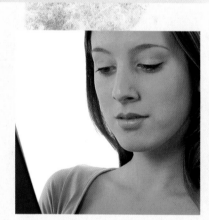

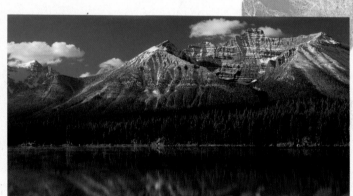

LOTUS BLOSSOM MEDITATION

Turn to the photograph of the beautiful lotus blossom (see *Nelumbo nucifera*) in the Flower and Plant Encyclopedia as a visual aid. Gaze at the picture with semifocused eyes so that the image appears hazy for a minute or two, then gently close your eyes and let your imagination drift. Create an environment around this blossom by perhaps visualizing it among many other flowers with the snow-capped mountains in the distance. Stay there for as long as you feel comfortable. Half open your eyes to look at the lotus flower again and make a mental note of how you feel and the impressions it is making upon you. Once the image is clear in your head, close your eyes again and visualize the blossom in your third eye (sixth chakra). After a while slowly open and focus your eyes. This meditation usually takes about 10 minutes. It will help to stimulate your imagination and activate your third eye, which enables you to see into other realms.

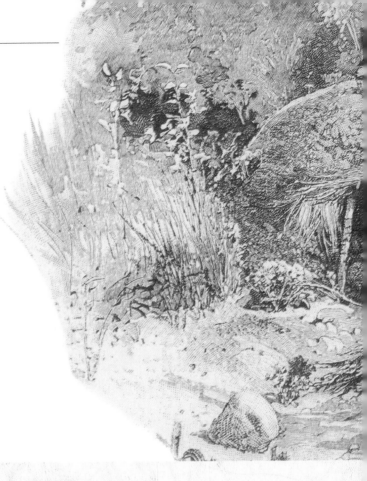

THE PURPOSE AND USE OF CEREMONY

A ceremony acts as a way in which we can express ourselves in a sacred manner. Performing certain rituals with reverence and respect brings purpose and focus to our intentions.

Some traditional ceremonies are highly theatrical, others can be very simple, yet each has the same objective. Carrying out your own ceremony provides the perfect means for honoring the gifts that the plant spirits can give.

People across the globe use ceremonies primarily as a means of reaffirming their connection with Mother Earth and to request the assistance of the spirit world. A ceremony may come from a vision that is handed down from generation to generation, or can be something you make up yourself.

The medicine wheel of the Native Americans is one of the oldest and most widely performed ceremonies. It symbolizes the circle of life and is used as a devise for obtaining spiritual knowledge, particularly about oneself, and for making

A CEREMONY OF THANKFULNESS

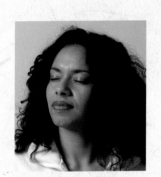

Performing a ceremony, no matter how simple, is a way of honoring this relationship. You will require some fresh flowers for this ceremony. Close your eyes and ask for guidance on which

In order to maintain an open and respectful relationship with the natural world and the nature spirits, it has always been considered polite and courteous to show our appreciation.

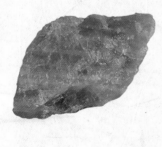

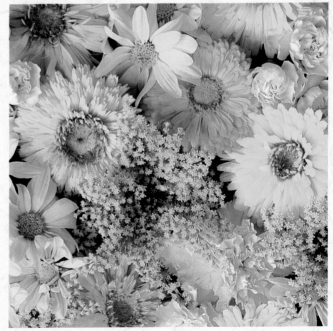

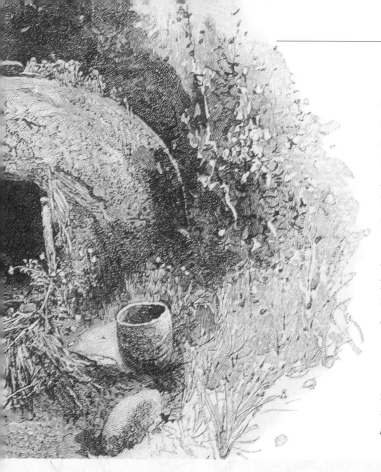

connections at different levels of reality. The wheel represents four stages of life – birth or renewal, growth, maturity, and death. These phases are linked to the south, west, north, and east as well as the four elements. Among Native Americans, certain plants are associated with each phase because their spirits are thought to assist with the various transitions in life.

Another ancient healing ceremony among Native Americans is that of the sweat lodge. Its primary purpose is purification of the spirit, and it has been used for centuries. Smoking herbs, such as sage and osha, traditionally form part of the ceremony.

LEFT *The sweat lodge was used by Native Americans to purify and heal the spirit.*

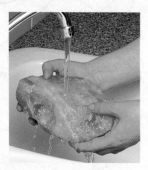

kind to use, then ask permission to gather them. Fill a crystal or glass bowl with spring water and float the freshly picked flowers on the surface.
Next choose a crystal –

rose quartz is good for this ceremony, but your favorite variety is just as effective. Before using this crystal it needs to be cleansed by holding it under running water for two minutes. The crystal will help to amplify your thoughts of thankfulness. Place this crystal in your garden or some quiet place in nature, such as at the foot of a favored tree, then place the

bowl with flowers beside it.
In your mind, thank nature and the plant spirits for the gifts they give so freely, and gently pour some of the water that the flowers are in over the crystal. This gives energy back to Mother Earth and shows thanks for her continued nurturing and support. If you wish to keep this as your special place of ceremony you could

leave the crystal there, perhaps even burying it in the earth to preserve the sacred energies of this place.

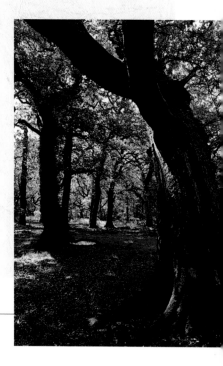

WORKING WITH PLANT SPIRIT MEDICINE

PLANT *spirit medicines are natural remedies inspired by the spirits of healing plants. Throughout history people discovered various ways to harness the life force or spirit energy of a plant.*

The medicines derived from plants take many different forms. They may be scented droplets of oils from flowers and leaves, liquids infused with flower petals, homeopathic dilutions of medicinal plants, or the smoke of smoldering herbs. What makes them special is their ability to heal on different levels – spiritual, emotional, mental, and physical. Some healers in the past may have discovered plants' different abilities by a process of trial and error but most shamans and medicine men and women claimed to have received their insights into the healing properties of plants through powerful dreams and visions.

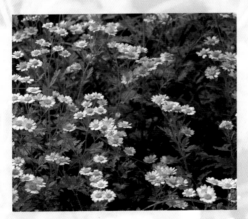

ABOVE *Different applications of plant remedies can be used to ease physical, mental, and spiritual problems.*

THE DISPENSATION OF KNOWLEDGE

To the ancients there was nothing mysterious about receiving knowledge in the form of visions and dreams. Such pearls of wisdom were regarded as gifts from the gods or spiritual domains. Among indigenous people it is generally accepted that the nature spirits guide them toward plants with medicinal properties and reveal ways they can be used as important healing medicines.

The forms in which plant remedies are used may vary from culture to culture. Among the Native Americans, for instance, there is an ancient healing tradition of using the smoke of plants such as tobacco, sage, and wormwood, which is uncommon in other parts of the world.

The Australian Aborigines are said to have discovered how to capture the healing essence of flowers through their dreamtime. Their ancient practice of sipping the dew drops that settle on the petals is embraced in the present-day form of flower essences and remedies. Down-to-earth ways of preparing medicinal plants and herbs to treat physical symptoms are common in every part of the world. The plants and their remedies were perfectly suited to the needs of the people who were using them.

Now we can all benefit from this synthesis of knowledge. When you turn to the Flower and Plant Encyclopedia you will discover more about the various forms in which plants are used for healing. The spirit of the rose, for instance, is encapsulated in its flower essence, perfumed or essential oil, and floral water. These are literally interpretations of the plant's spirit and reflect different aspects of its personality. You may choose to work with the plant spirit medicines singly or in combination to encourage healing at different levels of your being.

BELOW *An extensive collection of flowers and herbs can provide the remedy for many common ailments. Leaves, flowers, and oils can all be used.*

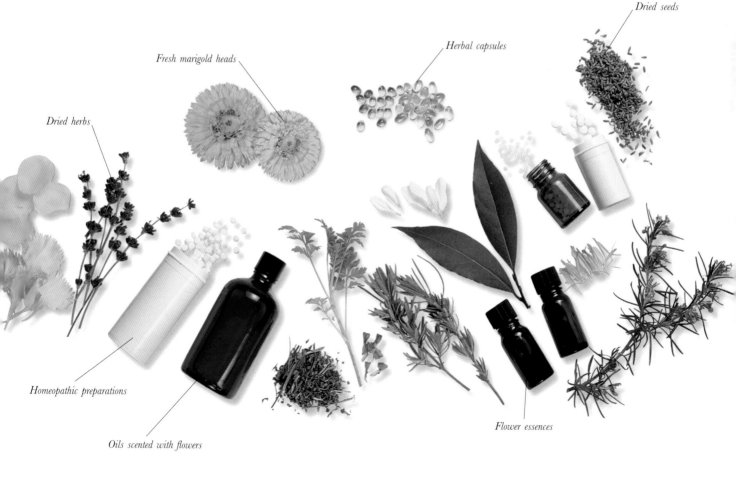

Dried seeds

Herbal capsules

Fresh marigold heads

Dried herbs

Homeopathic preparations

Oils scented with flowers

Flower essences

Flower Essences or Remedies

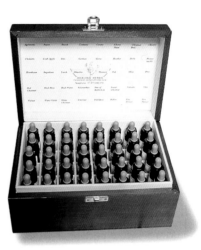

FLOWER ESSENCES ARE *the expression of the plant's spirit or deva. These subtle elixirs hold the unique energy patterns of flowers and encapsulate their healing qualities. They have long been used as remedies for various ailments of the spirit.*

RIGHT *A collection of flower essences.*

Flower essences are a form of liquid energy with amazing powers for uplifting the spirit and bringing relief from unsettling moods and emotions, such as fear, anxiety, guilt, anger, and melancholy, that often spring from the stress of modern living. Working with flower essences brings greater knowledge of oneself and evokes the power to face changes that make our lives more fulfilling. They are like guiding lights that inspire spiritual illumination.

HOW DO FLOWER ESSENCES HEAL?

The energy of every flower is unique and is captured within the flower essence. Being so similar in nature to our own subtle energies, the flower's energy harmonizes with them and can restore balance to the subtle anatomy. Stress, especially severe shock and trauma, are responsible for throwing our energy systems out of balance and putting our physical and emotional sides at risk. Areas where imbalance exists literally soak up the essences' healing energy. Some flower remedies act primarily at the emotional and mental levels, while many of the newer essences made from flowers such as roses, orchids, lotus, and other sacred blooms, affect us at the higher, spiritual level.

LEFT *Clematis is one of the plants used by Dr. Bach, who developed a healing system of flower remedies.*

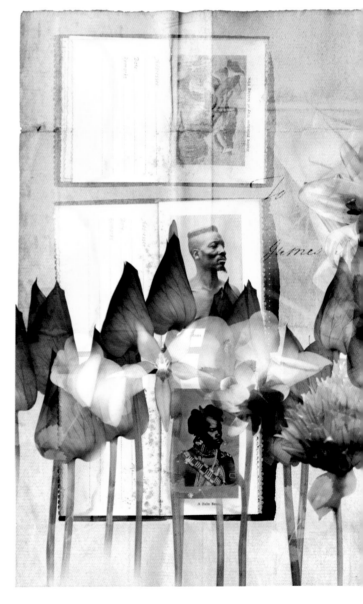

THE BIRTH OF FLOWER ESSENCES

The Australian Aborigines practiced one of the most ancient forms of flower essence therapy. Around 10,000 years ago, they were gathering dew-drenched flowers and placing them in their mouths. If the flowers were inedible, then they would simply sit among them. They believed the flowers could renew or revive a person's spirit. If someone was afraid, they would gain courage, if angry they would find peace, if sick they would become well again. It is thought that Native Americans, Minoans, and ancient Egyptians harnessed the healing powers of flowers in similar ways.

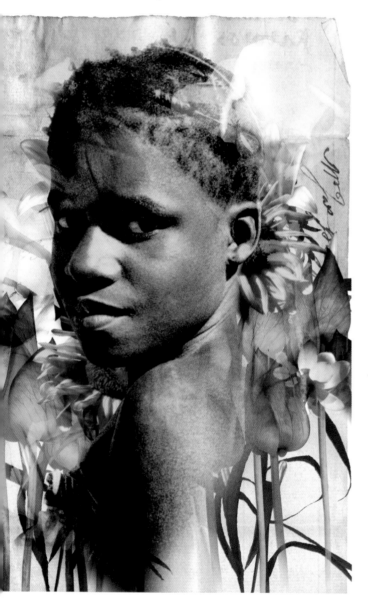

THE BACH REMEDIES

For many years, this healing art was lost in the mists of time. Then, in the 1920s, it was reborn through the work of Dr. Edward Bach, a respected Harley Street physician. Bach noted that stress underlies much illness and that personality influences how you respond to stressful events. In difficult times some people become irritable, while others have a propensity to become withdrawn or gloomy. Bach began his quest for a healing system that could help with the psychological aspect of illness. He intuitively turned to the flowers blossoming in the British countryside. Over a period of years, Bach scanned the fields and hedgerows looking for flowers that related to 12 key personality types. He then searched for other flowers that would relieve a further 26 states of mind. It is said that Bach would allow himself to succumb to negative moods and emotions, such as feelings of desperation and intense gloominess, then seek the flower that would restore his sense of well-being.

In recent years other people who communicate with the flower spirits or devas have prepared essences from a variety of other flowers, particularly those traditionally used in healing and regarded as having sacred qualities in their place of origin. Some flowers, especially those native to the Australian bush, Himalayan mountains, and Hawaii have a long history of being used as medicines. However, in more recent times, the range of plants used has grown ever larger. The newer flower essences are made from an extraordinarily diverse variety of flora, ranging from hedgerow and alpine flowers to exotic orchids, roses, and the blossoms of trees and fruits.

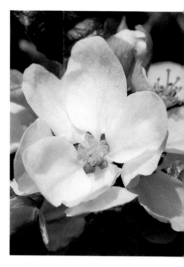

ABOVE *Apple blossom is one of the flowers used in modern forms of flower remedy.*

LEFT *Forms of flower therapy have been practiced around the world for thousands of years.*

HOW TO MAKE
FLOWER ESSENCES

Bach discovered that he could capture a flower's healing essence by floating freshly picked blooms in bowls of spring water and leaving them in the sunlight on a cloudless day. The "energized" water was then mixed with brandy, which acted as a preservative.

You could also try making your own flower essences. If possible, flowers destined for healing should be growing in wild places that are not often visited and are free from pollution. If taken from cultivated plants, it is important that the flowers are tended with loving care and without the use of chemical pesticides or fertilizers. An ideal remedy can be created from flowers you are instinctively drawn toward or those growing in your own garden. Only select ones that are in full bloom with an intense, vibrant color, remembering to ask permission to take them first. Rinse a glass or crystal bowl with salt water, then fill it with spring

LEFT Many wild flowers are protected species, but you can make flower essences from plants that have been grown organically.

water and float the flowers in the bowl for 2 to 3 hours in the sunshine. To make a mother tincture, use 50 percent flower water and 50 percent brandy. This is your own personal flower essence.

WORKING WITH FLOWER ESSENCES

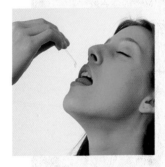

BY MOUTH
The traditional way of taking flower essences is to dilute them (10 drops to 2 tablespoons of pure spring water) and drop them under your tongue. This method harks back to the way ancient people would sip the dew drops from flowers and it seems to hasten their absorption. You could also add one or two drops to a glass of fruit juice or a cup of herbal tea.

ON THE SKIN
The energies of flower essences can be taken up through the skin. Good places to apply the drops

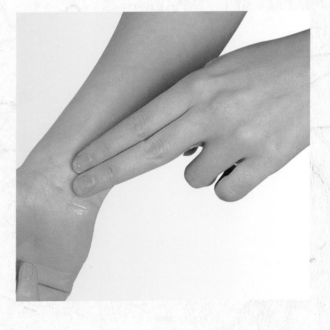

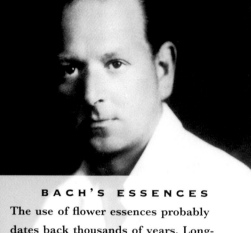

LEFT Choose good specimens of your favorite flowers to make your personal flower essence.

BELOW Experiment with a variety of essences to discover the ways in which they make you feel.

BACH'S ESSENCES

The use of flower essences probably dates back thousands of years. Long-forgotten in the West, they were rediscovered in the 1920s by Dr. Edward Bach. The success of his work, using British wild flowers, has inspired others to apply the techniques to flowers from all over the world.

are the forehead, lips, wrists, soles of feet, and palms of hands. You can also add a few drops to lotions, creams, ointments, oils, and compresses.

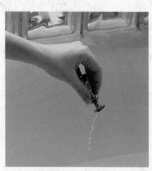

BATH THERAPY

Immerse yourself in the energies of flowers by adding a few drops of essence to your bath.

BODY SPLASH

Add about 7 drops of flower essence to a bowl of spring water and leave in the sun for a day, if possible. Splash this energized water over your

body and allow to dry naturally. Alternatively use an atomizer to spray the diluted essences onto your skin.

ROOM SPRAY

Spraying flower essences into the air is an excellent way to cleanse and revitalize the atmosphere of any room. Add 4–5 drops to a 10fl oz/300ml plant spray filled with still spring water and spray the mixture around the room every couple of hours.

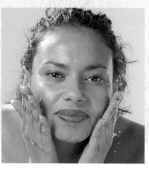

Sacred Smoke, Smudging, and Sacred Bundles

BURNING SACRED PLANTS *is a spiritual ritual practiced by religious peoples around the world. Smoke is thought to carry messages and prayers to the spirit world as well as containing the spirit of the plant itself. Burning sacred plants is a spiritual ritual practiced by religious peoples around the world.*

ABOVE *Burning resins produces fumes and aromas that play a central part in many spiritual rituals around the world.*

When beautiful blooms or aromatic tree resins are consumed by fire, their sweet perfumes are believed to please the gods or nature spirits. The smoke of burning herbs is traditionally seen as having the power to cleanse away any negative or harmful energies and to help people connect with the spirit world.

SACRED RESINS

Spiritual ceremonies have long been conducted in a haze of sacred smoke. The ancient Egyptians used aromatic blends including myrrh and frankincense to heighten spiritual awareness, promote meditative states, and appease their gods.

To the Mayan people of Central America the smoke of the sacred copal resins is used in healing ceremonies as well as to provide nourishment for their gods and the spirits of departed souls. The smoke is used by Mayan healers to enter a trancelike state and to scan their patient's body energy field. The smoke helps them to see where blockages exist. It then cleanses and raises the energetic vibrations to bring about healing.

Smudging is a traditional purification ritual performed by the Native Americans before any ceremony for healing or connecting with the spirits of nature. It is the act of burning a herb and washing oneself, the other participants, and the plants or ceremonial tools in its smoke. Smudging demarcates the ceremonial event in time, saying that from this point on what we do is sacred. It also serves to clear away any negative energy or vibrations and draws in those of a positive and healing nature.

PERFORMING A SMUDGING CEREMONY

It is a good idea to carry out a simple smudging ritual when you wish to attune to the spirits of plants or before a healing treatment, such as an aromatherapy massage or floral acupressure. Traditionally, a stone bowl is used as a container for the smudging herbs, but a clay bowl or mortar will do. The herbs commonly used by the Native Americans for smudging are sage, sweetgrass, cedar, tobacco, and wormwood. Small pieces of the herbs are placed in the bowl, lit with a coal or match, and then the flames are blown out so that the herbs smolder rather than burn. The smoke that rises is fanned with the hands or a feather, first toward the heart and

LEFT *Tree resins are used in many rituals throughout South America.*

HOW TO MAKE YOUR OWN SMUDGE STICK

A smudge stick is small bundle of herbs that you set alight, then blow out so that it smolders. You can use it like a broom to sweep around your body, as well as other places, to cleanse the

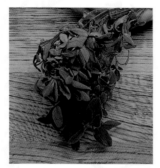

energies. You will need some sage picked just before it is about to bloom. Do this in a ceremonial way, asking for permission from the spirit of sage

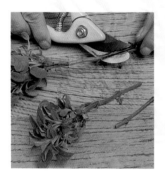

and laying an offering of loose tobacco leaves (as pure as possible) in the place of the sage as a token of thanks.

Cut the sage into 6in/15cm lengths and dry by hanging the bundle upside down in your kitchen. It can be

used alone or combined with cedar or lavender. In Celtic Druid tradition, mugwort, lavender, and sage were used together. When dry, bind the herbs together with red-colored thread – wool is good – wound up one way and criss-crossed down the other to make a mini-broom.

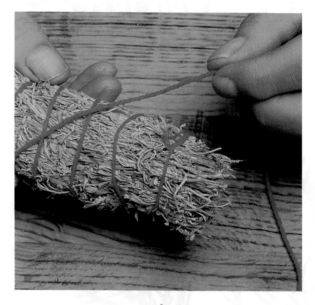

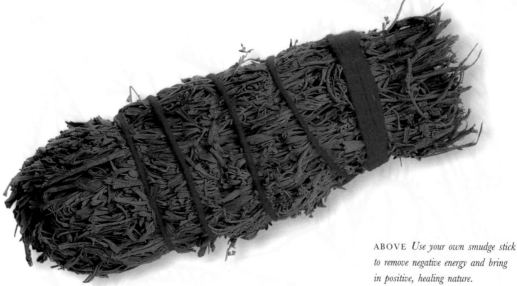

ABOVE *Use your own smudge stick to remove negative energy and bring in positive, healing nature.*

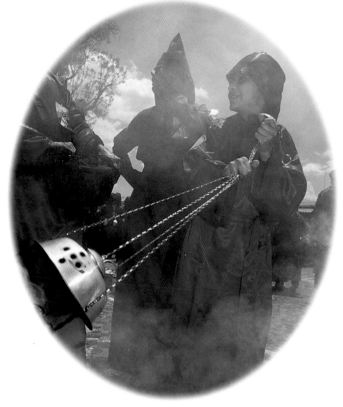

then above the head, helping the energy to move in the right direction. This form of washing with sacred smoke will clear away any negative feelings or influences while helping to restore energetic balance.

The bowl is then offered to the four corners of the earth. Plants considered sacred to certain directions are cedar and copal for the south, willow and sage for the west, sweetgrass for the north, and pine and tobacco for the east.

Smudging is also used to clear stagnant and negative areas in rooms or dwellings. It is good to start at the door and walk around the outskirts of the room gathering the old stale energy ahead of you, before moving back to the door and wafting any negative energy out through it. This will cleanse the area and encourage positive links with the spirit world.

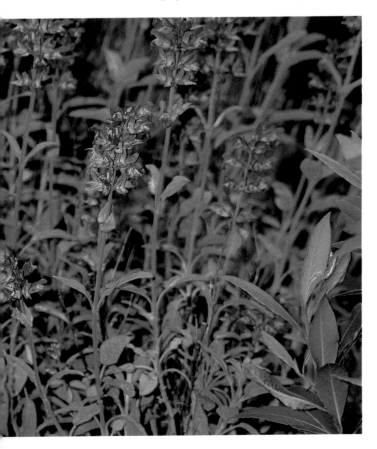

SACRED BUNDLES

Those who work with plant spirit medicines often carry a special collection of healing plants and herbs, for helping themselves and others, in a small bag or pouch. These sacred bundles can take several forms.

Native American tribal bundles are similar but hold ancient sacred objects over 100 years old. As keepers of tribal energy and power, the bags are often hidden or housed in special teepes. Traditionally they are made from animal skin such as buckskin or white deer skin. Ceremonial bundles contain objects that are used only in rituals for attuning to and connecting with the spirits.

There are healing bundles carried by medicine men and women that contain the tools of their trade. They are like a doctor's black bag but instead of pills and potions, they contain various stones, crystals, amulets, feathers, and herbs that are said to carry their power. Within a plant medicine person's bundle you will find sacred plants only.

A personal medicine pouch is a smaller version that can be worn around the neck for protection and to enhance fully your personal power.

HOW TO MAKE YOUR OWN SACRED MEDICINE POUCH

Choose some silk or a piece of soft leather and sew into a small bag or pouch. Into it you can place a healing bundle made with some sprigs of your favorite herb together with a little tobacco, which is a symbol of connection to spirit, and corn, for nurturing. You can also add small phials or bottles of helpful essential oils or flower remedies. Tie some silk or a beautiful cord around the bundle and keep it in a special place. Once a week take the bundle out, open it, and smudge it with your smudge stick to keep it energetically clean and clear.

RIGHT *A healing bundle can be made with herbs, tobacco, and essential oils or flower remedies, held within a soft leather pouch.*

Sacred Scents – Perfume and Aromatherapy

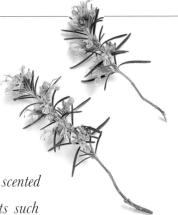

ABOVE Some plant perfumes are so strong that it is only necessary to squeeze a few drops from the plant.

T HE HEADY FRAGRANCE *of precious flowers, aromatic leaves, and richly scented resins has a potent influence on our mind, body, and spirit. To the ancients such perfumes possessed magical properties that could alter states of consciousness, induce tranquillity, arouse passions, and evoke sensuality.*

Some perfumes are so ethereal we can only enjoy their benefits by inhaling them. Other scents are contained in ultrafine oil drops that may be squeezed from the plant and used to enrich every aspect of our lives. Perfumes affect us in ways that we still do not fully comprehend; the exquisite fragrances of jasmine, rose, and sandalwood appear to uplift our spirits, while others subliminally affect our feelings, emotions, and patterns of behavior.

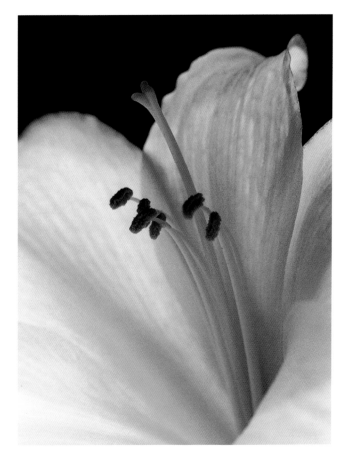

ABOVE The White Lily symbolizes purity of spirit. Its seductive aroma was used in magical ceremonies to heighten perceptions.

THE POWER OF PERFUME

The ancient Egyptians realized the potency of perfume. Blending aromas was the task of high priests who would create perfumes for different purposes, often spiritual. These scents were used in temples to evoke favors from the gods, to help the high priests contact the spirit world, and to create an atmosphere conducive to divinity. Each Pharaoh and his family had personalized perfumes designed to enhance their presence and personal power.

Nowadays we tend to wear perfume for its sensual appeal, but surrounding yourself with an aroma can bring other benefits. Scent can enhance your aura and subtly alter the way others perceive you. At the same time, a certain scent may bring feelings of inner calm, kindle the spark of life, or fire your passions.

THE PATHWAY OF PERFUME

Scent affects us primarily via our sense of smell. Aromatic molecules emitted by plants waft along our nasal passages and stimulate the ultrasensitive olfactory nerve endings. These nerves are unique for they enjoy direct access to an area of the brain known as the limbic system.

This region is concerned with intense emotional desires such as sex drive, hunger, thirst, and pleasure. The limbic system also seems responsible for many of the phenomena of altered states of consciousness, such as feelings of euphoria, loss of body awareness, sensations of floating or flying, and visual sensations such as seeing white or golden light, experiences common to those who meditate for long periods of time. This lends credibility to the ancients' long-established spiritual use of perfume.

HEALING SCENTS

Aromatherapy is the therapeutic use of aromatic plant extracts known as essential oils and can be traced back to the ancient Chinese, Indian, Hebrew, and Arab civilizations. However, it was the ancient Egyptians who perfected this art. They realized that many aromas are encapsulated in very fine oils that can be extracted from plants. These essential oils are sometimes referred to as the "soul" of a plant or as its hormones.

If you take a few leaves of lavender or rosemary and rub or squeeze them between your fingers you can smell the

essential oils. These aromatic oils occur in various different parts of a plant. Rose essential oil, for instance, comes from rose petals, lemon essential oil comes from lemon rind, while ginger essential oil comes from ginger root. Some plants, such as the orange tree, yield several different essential oils; one kind from its flowers, another from the rind of its fruits, and yet another from its leaves.

Each essential oil has its own distinctive aroma and therapeutic properties. Some have a general or stimulating effect on bodily functions. Most have a remarkable ability to promote the healing process and regenerate new skin tissue. Most are naturally antiseptic and will inhibit bacterial growth, making them valuable alternatives to conventional antibiotics.

BELOW *While walking through a grove of orange trees, the aroma of the blossoms therapeutically clears depression and lifts your spirit.*

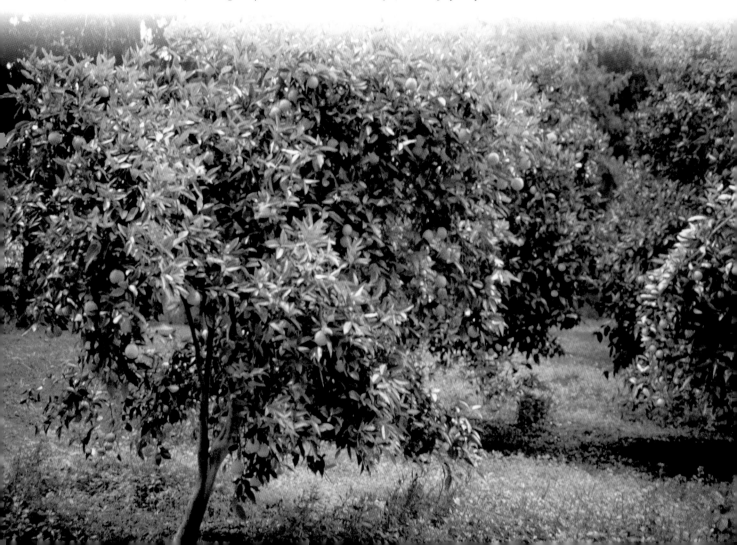

HOW TO WORK WITH PERFUMES AND ESSENTIAL OILS

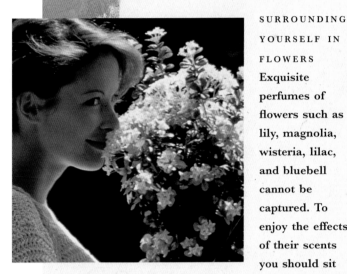

SURROUNDING YOURSELF IN FLOWERS

Exquisite perfumes of flowers such as lily, magnolia, wisteria, lilac, and bluebell cannot be captured. To enjoy the effects of their scents you should sit close to them or among them, preferably in a garden or natural setting. Their fine fragrances change the vibration of the energies around you and seem to enhance our perception of the energies or spirits around us. If you have ever walked among scented plants you will know how such floral perfumes can momentarily transport you to a "dreamier" world.

SCENTING THE AIR

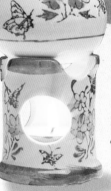

To enrich a room with aroma and create an atmosphere that is calming, energizing, meditative, clarifying, or sensual, place a few drops on a small clay dish and warm them with a candle (you can also buy vaporizers designed for this purpose). Use the more pungent antiseptic herbal essential oils, such as thyme, rosemary, and tea tree, to discourage the spread of infections, especially during the wintertime. To ease the symptoms of coughs and colds, a few drops can also be placed on a facial tissue for inhaling or dropped on the corners of your pillow.

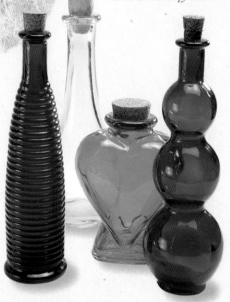

BELOW *Bath oils infused with herbs are a simple but effective way to treat yourself to an aromatherapy treatment.*

PERSONAL PERFUMES

Aromatherapeutic perfumes are made with the finest quality essential oils. Synthetic copies are chemical cocktails that do not have the same energy and vitality as the real thing. These synthetics tend to swamp rather than enhance your own subtle skin smell. Choose aromas that instinctively appeal to you. Keep your perfume simple. Using a single essence such as jasmine or rose is fine or try a combination of two or three harmonizing oils. Add about 30 drops of essential oil to 2 tablespoons of a fine vegetable oil and dab onto your pulse points.

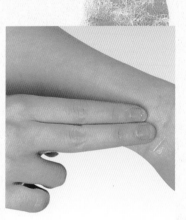

MASSAGE

Smoothing an aromatic oil over the skin combines the benefits of massage and aromatherapy. Select the essential oils for their therapeutic properties rather than for their aroma. They are taken up through the skin's pores, absorbed into the bloodstream, and attracted to areas where they are most needed. Add about **10** drops of essential oil to **2** tablespoons of carrier oil.

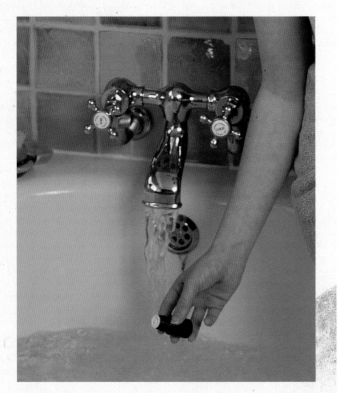

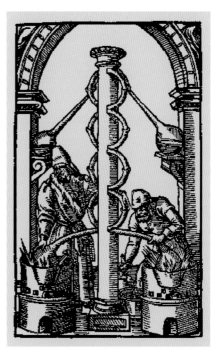

ABOVE *In alchemy there are three principles behind everything in creation – soul, spirit, and salt.*

IN THE BATH

An aromatherapy bath can be luxurious and therapeutic. It combines the benefits of inhaling the aroma and absorbing the essential oils through the skin. Add **10** drops of essential oils to your bath just before you've finished running it. Remember that some essential oils can irritate the skin; disperse them by adding to alcohol or to a tablespoon of milk before adding to the water.

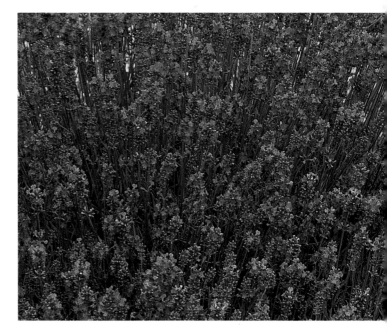

ABOVE *Lavender is the best known "nose herb," valued for its fresh calming fragrance. Its oil composes the mind and clears buildup of nervy stress and unexpressed emotions.*

Plant and Flower Preparations

THROUGHOUT HISTORY AND *across all cultures people have found various ways of distilling the healing essence of plants to make medicines. Methods for preparing the leaves, petals, stems, roots, and barks of plants have been handed down from generation to generation and are still widely used.*

ABOVE *The foxglove is just one plant that was used as a source of medical remedy.*

Healing plants may be simmered in water to make therapeutic drinks or dissolved in alcohol to create more potent medicinal liquids. Fresh leaves and flowers may be wrapped around the skin or steeped in oil and milks to make soothing body balms. Remedies made from basic plant matter work wonders for relieving the physical symptoms of illness.

THE OLDEST MEDICINES

Plants are our most ancient form of medicine. Archeological evidence found at Shanidar in Iraq shows that Neanderthal man was using healing plants about 6,000 years ago. The very same plants discovered at this site are still used by the tribes living in this area, suggesting they are as valuable today as they were then.

Virtually every culture has a healing tradition that relies on plants and herbs. For centuries people have found the medicines they need growing close by. In arid desert regions we find plants such as aloe vera whose gel has the power to soothe and heal burns inflicted by the sun. In contrast, willow (*Salix* spp.), a tree whose bark yields a pain-relieving substance called salicin that eases rheumatic aches and pains, springs up in damp, water-logged areas of the Northern Hemisphere.

Our early ancestors knew nothing of chemistry and pharmacology. They relied on their intuition and powers of observation to guide them toward plants that could relieve their ills. Watching animals, who know instinctively which plants to look for when they are sick, they learned of nature's healing powers. Their discoveries were augmented by sacred knowledge passed on by those who could sense the healing vibrations of plants.

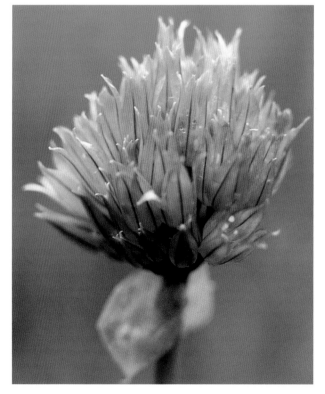

AN EXPRESSION OF SPIRIT

Many indigenous people believe a plant gives clues to its healing powers in its flowers, coloration, growth patterns, and even habitat. For instance, in West Africa people think a spotted leaf will help to treat a spotted skin. This principle of similarity was very popular in sixteenth-century Europe. Paracelsus, a Swiss physician and mystic, was one of its leading proponents and embellished the idea of sympathy

LEFT *Wild garlic is a well-known healing plant.*

between plant and illness in the Doctrine of Signatures. A classic example is the foxglove (*Digitalis purpurea*) whose purple flowers, symbolic of blood, bear a resemblance to an open heart. We know foxglove yields a chemical called digitalis, used for treating heart problems. Look closely at camomile and we find subtle hints of its ability to soothe nervous digestive problems. Its flower-heads form a pattern similar to that of the stomach's secretory cells, while its thin wavy leaves remind us of what nerve fibers look like.

ABOVE *Many plants can be applied directly to the skin in a compress.*

BELOW *The intricate patterns formed by the twigs and branches of a tree, such as the willow, are reminiscent of the veins and nerves of the human body.*

THE POTENCY OF PLANTS

We often assume that because plants are "natural" they are also gentle and safe, which is not always true. Healing plants often owe their medicinal properties to chemicals such as alkaloids, steroids, and glycosides with potent pharmacological effects. Many such compounds have inspired our modern medicines. Quinine, for example, is one of 25 alkaloids found in the bark of the cinchona tree native to South America. The

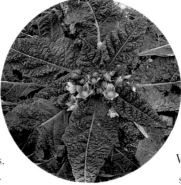

ABOVE *Long associated with magic and mysticism, a mandrake was used to engender shamanic trances.*

bark is traditionally brewed into a tea by the Native South Americans who have drunk this concoction for hundreds of years. The quinine alkaloid turned out to be an effective anti-malarial treatment. There are countless other examples. Codeine and morphine are derived from the opium poppy (*Papaver somniferum*), while the preanesthetic hyoscine and motion-sickness drug hyosyamine both come from mandrake (*Mandragora officinarum*). Indeed the plant world still holds the greatest promise for discovering future medicines.

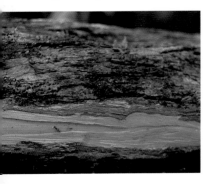

ABOVE *The bark of the cinchona tree is a source of quinine.*

To make modern medicines, pharmaceutical companies isolate and reproduce the most active chemical substances from such plants. In nature, plants contain an abundance of different chemicals, enzymes, and nutrients, which may all work together in some as yet unexplained way. Herbalists and phytotherapists believe the whole plant is therapeutically superior to any isolated ingredients or chemically synthesized analogues.

Nowadays, we demand medicines that bring rapid relief from troubling complaints such as headaches. But swallowing a pill in a hurry, even if it is a herbal one, is at odds with the sacred way of healing. To the tribal medicine man or shaman, the plant material is merely the vehicle through which the spirit heals. The way plants are made into remedies and used is part and parcel of the healing process. It

begins with the simple ritual of preparation. Making a simple tisane connects you with the spirit of the plant and focuses your mind on the intention of healing. Set aside a quiet time to use or apply your plant remedies and contemplate their purpose. When sipping your herbal tisane, inhale its scent and savor its taste. Note any changes, no matter how subtle, in how you feel after using the remedy.

WORKING WITH PLANT MEDICINES

The medicinal parts of plants, herbs, and flowers can be prepared in many different ways. Before you begin, however, be sure of your plant's identity. Some plants look very similar and it is easy to make mistakes, especially if you are gathering plants from the wild. For your own safety, never pick or use a plant unless you are absolutely sure of its identity. It may be wise to obtain fresh herbs and other plants from

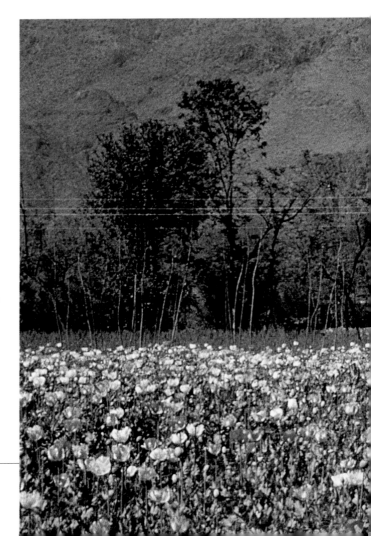

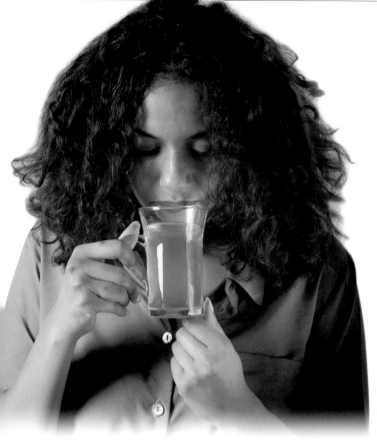

a specialist who grows them without the use of fertilizers or pesticides until you become really familiar with their appearance, aroma, taste, and any other distinguishing features.

When sufficiently confident to gather the plants yourself there are a few things to bear in mind. Try to avoid picking plants that are extremely dry or damp. Choose a clear sunny day to go gathering and take only the healthiest looking plants or flowers. Remember to give thanks to the plant and perhaps perform a simple ceremony.

When preparing your own plant medicines, use just one variety of plant or herb at a time rather than mixing them. As with any medical prescription, an expert knowledge of the chemical and botanical compatibility of different plants is required if you are to blend the right plants together in the correct proportions.

LEFT *Don't make your own plant remedies unless you are confident that you have built up your knowledge of plants and their powers.*

BELOW *A field of opium poppies – a field of dreams.*

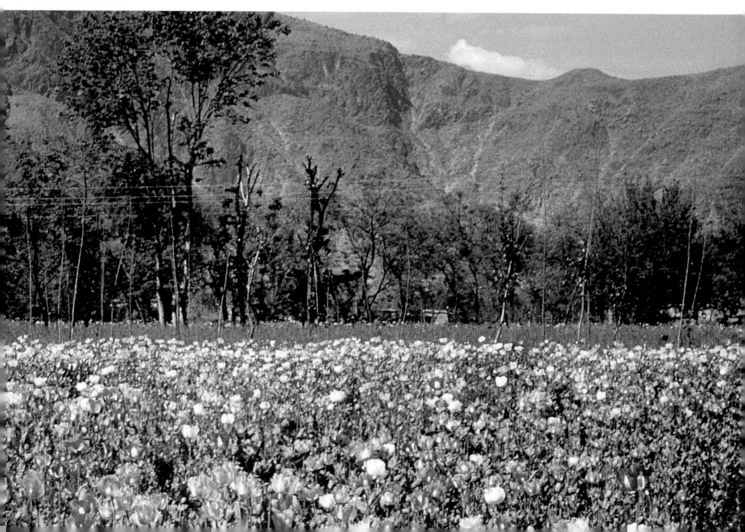

PLANTS AS MEDICINAL FOODS

In the early days plants were taken in their crudest form – you simply chewed upon a leaf, some bark, or a root. Some leafy plants, especially herbs, are best taken in their fresh, raw state because they contain enzymes, nutrients, and vitamins that can be destroyed by heating. Other more fibrous plants and roots, such as ginger, require some preparation and cooking to kindle their activity.

In China and other Eastern countries, there is an ancient tradition of using medicinal plants and herbs in cooking as a means of maintaining a sense of inner balance and harmony. Conditions linked to a predominance of yin are relieved with soups and stews made from plants and foods with prevalent yang properties.

FOODS WITH YANG PROPERTIES

陽

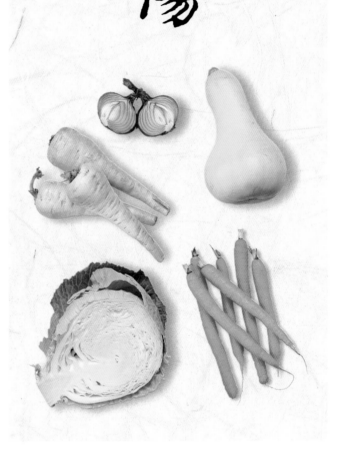

FOODS WITH YIN PROPERTIES

陰

One way to enjoy the therapeutic benefits of plants and herbs on a daily basis is to sprinkle them into your salads and to use them in your cooking. Grow a few of your favorite herbs in a window box so that you always have fresh ones at hand when you're cooking.

DRYING PLANTS, HERBS, AND FLOWERS

By drying your favorite plants you can have a supply of them all year round. Careful drying preserves most of the active ingredients but the fungi and bacteria that can cause a plant to ferment or rot are deprived of the moisture they need to flourish. If dried properly, plants should retain about 10 percent of their moisture content so that they maintain a sense of freshness and do not crumble in your hands.

PLANT PREPARATIONS

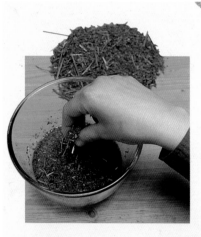

TINCTURES

Tinctures are alcoholic solutions containing the active principles of herbs and plants. Preparation is a technical procedure best performed by a professional herbalist or pharmacist. Essentially, ground or chopped herbs are left to steep in alcohol for about three weeks, then a small quantity of glycerine is added before the mixture is strained and stored in air-tight containers. Tinctures tend to be stronger volume for volume than infusions or decoctions.

The usual dose is 10–20 drops taken in a wineglass of water. If you want to avoid the alcohol, add to just-boiled water and let stand until tepid.

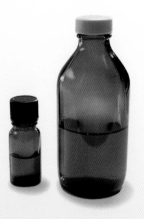

INFUSIONS

The most familiar way of making a tea from flowers, leaves, and green stems is by infusion. Use 1 tablespoon of dried herbs to 20fl oz/600ml of water or 1 heaped teaspoon per cup.

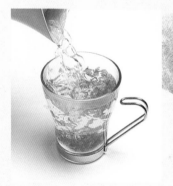

When using fresh herbs, you can double the quantity of herb. Place the herbs in a pot or cup, pour boiling water on them, cover, and let stand for about 4 minutes for a tisane, up to 10 minutes for a stronger infusion. Strain and drink either hot or cold, and sweetened with honey to taste. Hot infusions tend to encourage perspiration, so they are helpful for treating colds, flu, and fever.

DECOCTIONS

For harder parts of plants such as berries, seeds, woody roots, and barks you will need to make a decoction. Use the same quantities as recommended for infusions, although you may need to add a little more water to allow for evaporation. Place the herb or herbs in a saucepan and pour the water on them. Bring to a boil and then simmer for 3 to 5 minutes before straining. Use a glass, ceramic or enamel pan, not an aluminum one.

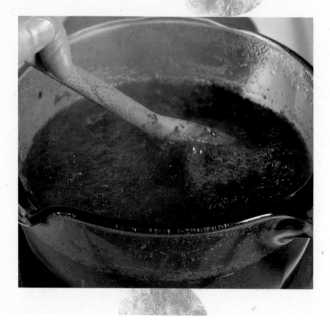

PLANT PREPARATIONS

COMPRESSES

Like therapeutic bandages, compresses bring the plant's active components into direct contact with the skin. To make a compress, use a clean cloth (an absorbent cotton pad or some linen or gauze will do) and soak it in a hot infusion or decoction. While still as warm as possible, place the compress on the affected area and cover with a piece of woolen material. The warmth will encourage the absorption of the therapeutic principles. Remove the compress when it is cold.

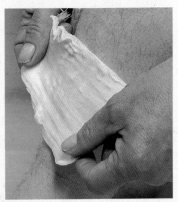

POULTICE

A poultice is the most primitive form of compress and involves using either fresh or dried herbs. Apply the bruised leaves, petals, or crushed root of the fresh plant to the skin, either directly or between thin layers of gauze. When using dried herbs first make a paste by adding hot water and mixing with soothing, slippery elm powder as a binder, then apply in the same way as a compress.

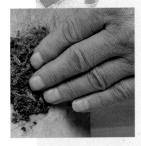

MUSLIN BAGS

Place either fresh or dried flowers, leaves, stems, or roots in a small bag of gauze or muslin, immerse in hot water, and then place on the area needing treatment. Cover the bag with a piece of wool or flannel and leave in place for 20 to 30 minutes. The same bags can be hung under warm running water to make a therapeutic bath. While bathing you can use them to rub over the skin.

FLORAL CREAMS

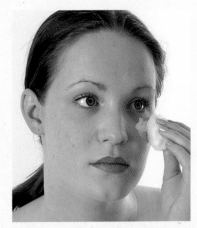

To make your own sweet-scented beauty treatment cream, gather a handful of fresh flowers in full bloom and add them to a saucepan containing 10fl oz./ 300ml of buttermilk. Heat gently for 30 minutes without allowing the mixture to boil. Remove from the heat and let it steep for 3 hours. Strain off the blossoms, reheat, and add 1oz/25g of set honey. Allow to cool and store in a dark-colored jar in the refrigerator.

PLANT OILS

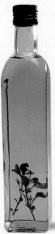

These plant-infused oils are very useful for smoothing over large areas of skin. Place a handful of the fresh or dried plant into a bottle containing 20fl oz./ 600ml of cold-pressed, virgin olive oil and leave to stand in the sun for 2–3 weeks. Filter and remove any water that has collected on the surface. You will need to keep this oil in a dark-colored bottle.

SYRUPS

Syrups offer a means of making bitter-tasting plants more palatable. They are particularly good for children and make soothing treatments for conditions such as coughs and bronchitis, sore

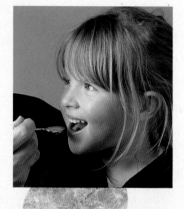

throats, tonsillitis and laryngitis. Place 4oz./100g of dried or fresh herbs in 2pt./1l of water. Boil for 1 minute and let the mixture stand for 2 to 3 days, then press and filter. Add raw cane sugar at a ratio of 1lb/500g to 2pt./1l of infusion. Once all the sugar has dissolved, pour into a tinted bottle and keep cool in the refrigerator.

FLORAL WATERS

When flowers such as rose, lavender, and orange flowers are distilled to make essential oils, an aqueous liquid is formed that contains the water-soluble parts of the flower. These distillates are referred to as floral waters. In the past they were highly prized as beauty treatments and have a wonderfully refreshing and toning effect on the skin. Some floral waters can also be added to a cup of warm water to create soothing, therapeutic drinks.

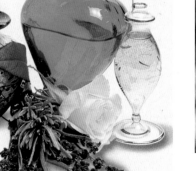

ALCHEMY AND PLANTS

Alchemists believe that in order to get the maximum benefit from a plant its three principles must be extracted: the essential oil, or soul; the alcohol-soluble compounds, or the spirit; and the alkaline salts extracted from the ashes of the plant, or the body. These principles are then recombined to make an alchemical elixir.

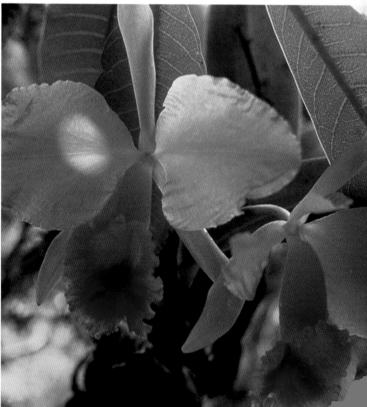

ABOVE *Orchid oil is highly valued as a skin rejuvenator. As a flower essence a couple of drops added to floral water can lend a spiritual element to a spritz.*

Homeopathic Plant Preparations

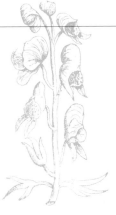

HOMEOPATHY IS A *form of spirit medicine that harnesses minute quantities of healing plants. Like flower essences, homeopathic remedies are plant preparations with the power to revitalize our life force and restore a sense of inner balance and tranquillity.*

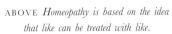

ABOVE *Homeopathy is based on the idea that like can be treated with like.*

When making homeopathic medicines, tinctures made from flowers, leaves, roots, stems, and bark are diluted time and time again until little of the original substance remains. What lingers is the molecular imprint of its active ingredients.

MORE IS LESS

The principles of homeopathy are based on an ancient Greek doctrine that says "let like be cured with like." Present-day homeopathy was developed by Samuel Hahnemann (1755–1843), a German physician. He discovered that a remedy made from cinchona tree bark (used to

ABOVE *Christian Friedrich Samuel Hahnemann, discoverer of homeopathy.*

treat malaria) when taken by a healthy person triggered the same sort of symptoms that it usually relieves. He also found that minuscule amounts of the same substance could then switch off the symptoms again. In Hahnemann's further research, the same principles held true. He noticed that the more he diluted his tinctures, the more effective they became. Often no trace of the original substance could be found in the actual remedy. This meant potentially toxic plants with medicinal properties such as deadly nightshade (*Atropa belladonna*) could be made into safe yet effective homeopathic remedies.

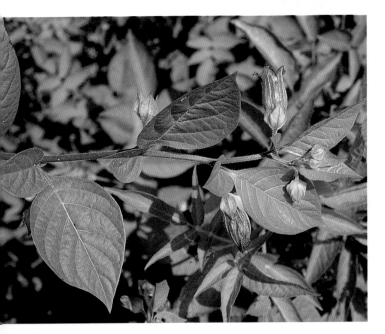

HOW DO HOMEOPATHIC REMEDIES WORK?

Like flower essences, homeopathic remedies seem to act primarily at an energetic level. Hahnemann believed in a life-giving energy and suggested that this vital force continually adjusts throughout our life to keep us healthy and balanced, physically, mentally, and spiritually. The symptoms of illness are signs that the body is coping with some kind of stress. The homeopathic remedies work by stimulating the vital force, helping the body to deal with the stress and restoring a state of equilibrium. A wide variety of homeopathic medicines with which to achieve this are now available.

LEFT *Some plants that are potentially poisonous can be used safely as homeopathic remedies.*

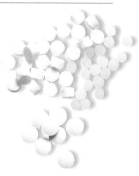

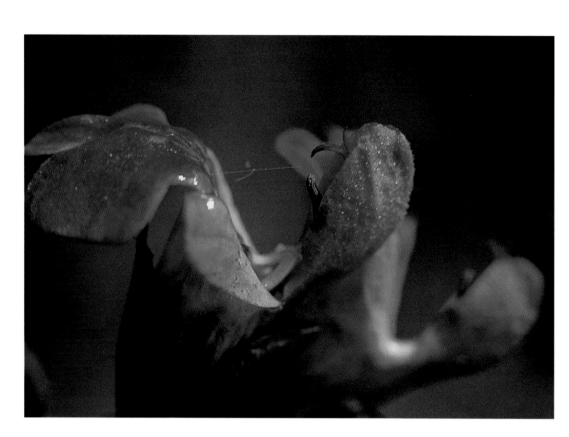

ABOVE *Homeopathic remedies are easily contaminated, so handle them as little as possible.*

LEFT *Sage is used for night sweats, coughs and to dry up breast milk.*

HOW TO CHOOSE AND USE THESE REMEDIES

Selecting the most appropriate homeopathic remedy means finding the best match for your symptoms. A cough, for instance, can take various different forms. It may be dry and rasping or loose and rattling. Physical symptoms are also usually accompanied by noticeable changes in emotion and behavior. Alterations in appetite, food preferences, moods, and mental state should all be noted when choosing the correct homeopathic remedy. Every plant-inspired remedy, therefore, will treat all the aspects of disharmony – emotional, mental, and physical.

Homeopathic remedies are taken individually so you can gage effectiveness. If you are new to homeopathy, opt for the lower dilutions (the least potent) such as the 6c, 12c, and 30c. Only use the 30c when you are sure you have found the remedy that matches the major symptoms.

Avoid handling the remedies unnecessarily. Tip them into the lid of the bottle, then pop them on your tongue. Never put remedies that have fallen onto the floor or elsewhere back into the bottle because they will contaminate the others. The remedies should be stored in a cool dark place with their tops screwed on tightly, away from strong-smelling substances such as perfumes and essential oils. Similarly avoid using peppermint-flavored toothpaste or drinking coffee when taking the remedies. For best effects avoid eating or drinking anything (except water) for 10 to 20 minutes before and after. Such external influences will interfere with the carefully prepared homeopathic remedies.

The first homeopathic hospital in London, England, opened in 1850. Although interest declined in the early twentieth century, the popularity of homeopathy has increased over recent years and it is now more widely used than ever.

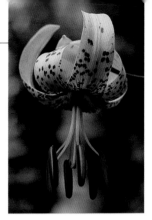

Using the Plant Spirit Medicines

T HE MOST COMPLETE *form of healing comes from working with plants in all their therapeutic forms. When used in combination the various preparations will complement each other and help to restore and enhance a total sense of well-being.*

ABOVE *A feminine flower, as a flower essence tiger lily brings inner peace and harmony to relationships.*

Specific plant preparations affect different aspects of our being. The reason for using various preparations together is that each augments the therapeutic benefits of the other.

Flower essences are drawn to particular areas of the subtle anatomy and exert a healing influence on the aura to affect us at the spiritual and emotional levels. The perfume of flowers and their essential oil influence our mood, behavior, and feelings by gaining direct access to the subconscious region of our brain. Applied to the skin, essential oils are taken into the physical body and influence various physiological processes. Infusions, tisanes, and floral waters exert their soothing influence at the physical level from both within and without.

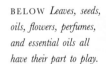

BELOW *Leaves, seeds, oils, flowers, perfumes, and essential oils all have their part to play.*

ABOVE *The heady perfume of the lily floods the senses with a warm and exotic aroma.*

Plant remedies designed to tackle physical upsets often trigger unpleasant emotions and sensations, a form of toxic release that must occur before the body can return to a state of balance. When using homeopathic remedies, a "healing crisis" may occur when the symptoms get worse before they get better. The side-effects may be eased by taking the flower essence derived from the same plant that created the homeopathic remedy – for instance camomile flower essence in conjunction with camomilla homeopathic remedy. Together they seem to speed the healing process.

FLORAL PREPARATIONS

HOW TO MAKE A FLORAL SPRITZ

Combine the essential oils and flower essences of your favorite flowers and plants to create body

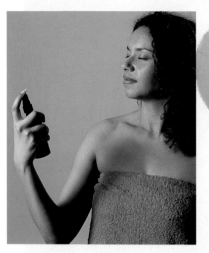

sprays that work wonders for re-balancing the subtle anatomy and aura. The following recipe is a special blend designed to cleanse and revitalize the aura.

Take a 5fl. oz./ 100ml atomizer or pump-action spray bottle and pour in 2 teaspoons of vodka. Add 2 drops each of the following pure essential oils: lavender, frankincense, geranium, and cedar. Replace the top and shake vigorously to disperse the essential oils, then add 2 drops each of the following flower essences: aloe vera, lotus, orchid, and yarrow. Fill the bottle with spring water and shake well once more. Spray your face, around your head, and, at arm's length, over your body to keep the energy field refreshed and protected.

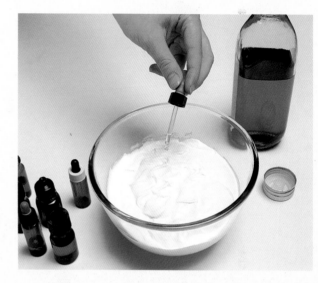

CALMING AND REJUVENATING CREAM

Into a glass bowl, mix a 1lb/500g tub of aqueous cream with 1 tablespoon of olive oil. Add 5 drops of each of the following essential oils: jasmine, rose, camomile, and frankincense. Next, stir in 5 drops of each of the following flower essences: lotus, orchid, and aloe vera.

FLORAL ACUPRESSURE

Floral acupressure is when flower essences are applied directly to certain acupressure points. A typical example would be using emotionally calming and soothing flower essences such as camomile, angelica, rosemary, or echinacea on the Pericardium 7 or Darling point (situated at the center of the main crease on the wrist), which is traditionally worked

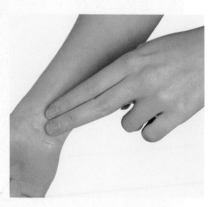

upon to relieve emotional anxiety, frazzled nerves, and a troubled mind.

FLORAL BEAUTY LOTION

You can also make your own complexion creams by using a blend of flower essences and essential oils. For a very simple preparation, blend rose essential oil and rose flower essence together.

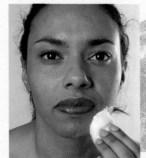

When you become more familiar with the different plants you can use them to create a cream that is specially designed to suit your particular needs.

THE OLDEST HEALING ART

THE PURSUIT OF *spiritual perfection can be traced back to the dawn of civilization. Thousands of years ago wise people realized* that spiritual qualities such as compassion, wisdom, and understanding were inextricably linked to feeling truly content and at peace with life.

The ancients saw happiness as an enlightened state, and their healing arts aimed to promote a sense of spiritual as well as emotional and physical well-being. In trees, plants, and flowers they saw divine qualities that could inspire this form of healing.

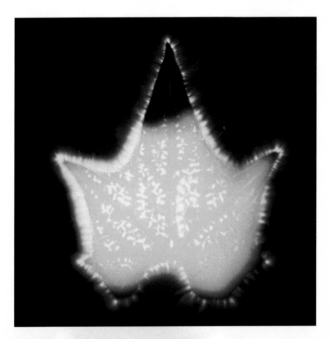

ABOVE *Spiritual enlightenment and physical health are inextricably linked.*

QUEST FOR SPIRITUAL PERFECTION

As far back as we are able to delve in history, people have worshiped nature and connected it to a higher spiritual reality or divinity. One hundred thousand years ago, Neanderthals used flowers in their burial ceremonies, and the earliest cave paintings suggest primitive people felt that animals, rocks, and trees possessed spirits. A common thread running through all religions is a belief in a divine force or spirit that fashioned everything in nature. From the earliest times, people strove to connect with the sacred as a means of rising above mundane reality.

Hinduism, Buddhism, Taoism, and other ancient religions proposed that matter and material creation had to be transcended in order to attain union with the greater and truer God whose domain was pure spirit. Among the ancient Egyptians and other spiritual people we discover a common quest to integrate matter with spirit as a means of bringing heaven down to earth. The pursuit of spiritual perfection and self-purification was felt to hold the key to a better life.

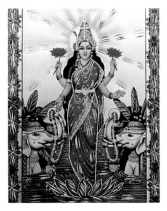

ABOVE *Lakshmi, the Hindu goddess of wealth, beauty, and good luck.*

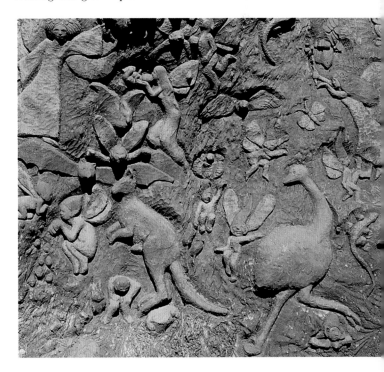

ABOVE *The Christian faith has its version of paradise in the story of Adam and Eve in the Garden of Eden.*

BELOW *Symbolism from nature is revealed in this "fairy tree" in the Fitzroy Garden, Melbourne.*

flavor that bloomed all year round bringing happiness to whoever wished for it yet losing its splendor in the hands of the sinful. Legends has it that in Lemuria all beings appeared as shimmering, ethereal entities, and people could "see" the healing energies of plants and flowers.

RETURN TO PARADISE

Myths and religions from around the world refer to a land of beauty and splendor where the gods or spiritually enlightened people dwelt. This heavenly place is referred to as Lemuria or Mu by the Native Americans, as Dilmun in Mesopotamian legends, as the Garden of Indra situated on Mount Meru in the confines of Kashmir in Indian tradition, and as the Garden of Eden in the Bible.

Within these magical gardens, watered by springs and rivulets, were luminous flowers and trees bearing fruits that conferred divine wisdom and immortality. In the Garden of Indra grew the "paridjata," a flower with every scent and

ANCIENT SUPER-RACE?

Although they spring from the minds of people who lived thousands of miles apart, the various descriptions of paradise show amazing similarities. Did such a land exist at some time in our prehistory? Evidence of an extremely ancient civilization populated by intelligent people with an amazing knowledge of astronomy and the natural word is beginning to emerge. These people appear to have aligned their temples and sacred sites to certain constellations in the sky in an attempt to reflect heaven on earth. It is claimed that vestiges of this civilization can be traced to the pyramids at Giza, the temples of Angkor in Cambodia, and the Nazca lines in Peru.

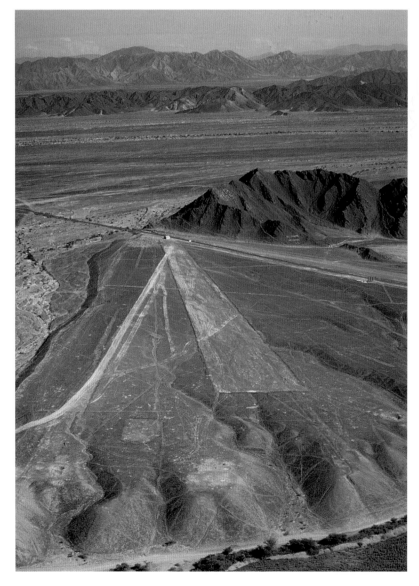

The collapse of this civilization may have occurred when a meteorite struck earth and floods engulfed the land. Did some survive this cataclysm and eventually come to settle in other lands, bringing with them their wisdom and beliefs? If so, the age-old belief in the sacred qualities of certain trees, plants, and flowers may be rooted in such a time.

THE TREE OF LIFE

Many traditions speak of a "tree of life" that links heaven and earth. It is rooted in the underworld yet its branches reach up to the heavens, symbolizing humankind's striving for perfection. The Scandinavians have Yggdrasil, an evergreen ash tree that, in its mythological form, represents the entire world. Its trunk represents the central axis of the universe, and from beneath its roots bubble the rivers or waters of wisdom. In Siberian mythology, the axis of the universe is a birch, larch, or golden oak tree that connects heaven to earth. The ancient earth goddess dwells in the tree itself or by its roots; the souls of unborn children live in its branches, like birds; while the sun and moon take their seats near the top.

To the Mayan people of Mexico, the ceiba tree, found at the entrance to the sacred pyramids at Tikal, is a model for their sacred world tree. Similarly the Mayan king was said to be a human embodiment of the ceiba as the central axis of the world, while the white flowers were the souls of his people.

Today Muslims still kneel to pray on carpets embroidered with trees of life, a powerful symbol of ascent and salvation.

The tree of life, then, represents a vision of eternal life. Just as a tree bears flowers or fruits every spring, so person's soul is born and reborn over and over again. This concept ties in neatly with the age-old pursuit of spiritual perfection.

LEFT *Nazca lines in Peru are said by shamans to be land-maps created by star beings that landed on earth.*

From a spiritual perspective it may be reasoned that if there is a purpose to life, it is surely to gain wisdom, knowledge, and enlightenment. It was thought that such spiritual endeavors purified the soul and in doing so ultimately brought release from the endless cycle of regeneration. In other words, spiritual perfection was the key that everyone was striving for, not only to feeling happy in this life, but also to attaining immortality and dwelling eternally in paradise.

IMAGE OF THE GODS

A belief in the sacred nature of certain trees, plants, and flowers dates from the earliest times. The earliest symbol of the sacred tree or plant can be traced back to the Akkadians who dwelt in the city of Eridu, which flourished on the shores of the Persian Gulf between 4,000 and 3,000 B.C.E. The rudimentary image may be a palm, pomegranate, cypress, or vine, yet each is the embodiment of a god.

In the Hindu Atharva-Veda, the tree *Ficus religiosa*, commonly known as the peepul, is referred to as the seat of the gods. It was the abode of the Hindu Triad, comprising Brahma, Vishnu, and Shiva. It was revered for its life-giving, magical, and medicinal properties.

LEFT *Sacred plants are often depicted on carvings adorning religious edifices.*

THE TREE OF LIFE

The concept of the tree of life is common to mythologies in the Old World and the New. The Cabala, the esoteric spiritual tradition within Judaism, uses the basic structure of the tree of life with its fruit, the ten Sefirot or spheres of consciousness, as a paradigm for spiritual perfection.

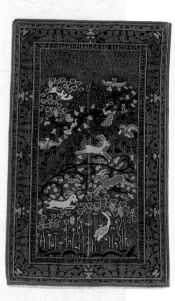

RIGHT *This carpet shows a flourishing tree of life.*

To the ancient Egyptians, the green sycamores that flourish along the Nile were considered sacred; the district around Memphis contained several trees believed to be inhabited by detached doubles of Nut, the sky goddess, and Hathor the earth goddess. The great Egyptian god Osiris originally took the form of the acacia tree. Egyptians believed the lotus was the first living thing to appear upon the earth. When the petals unfurled, the supreme god Amon, or Ptah, was revealed to them. In Hindu mythology, the supreme deity, Brahma, also emanated from a golden lotus.

ABOVE *The lotus – the most spiritual flower.*

SOMA

It was generally felt that the divine qualities of these sacred plants could be imbibed by simply being in their presence as well as using preparations made from them. An Indian spiritual teaching known as the Rig-Veda tells us that a plant called soma, regarded as a god, was employed by the Vedic and Avestan priests for its sacred functions. This life-giving plant growing in the mountains was said to bestow eternal life upon humankind. It gave men strength, poets inspiration, brought renewed virility to the aged, and ultimately evoked a blissful immortality. "We have drunk soma, we have become immortal, we have gone to the light, we have found the gods."

GATEWAY TO THE GODS

Among many indigenous peoples, visionary plants were deemed sacred because they appeared to open the door to a different reality. These divine medicines were thought to remove the barriers between humankind and the realm of gods and spirits who are the keepers of sacred wisdom. Visionary plants are an essential feature of shamanism in many regions. Modern research reveals that powerful chemicals in most sacred plants are capable of producing dramatic and often profound changes in perception. Colors are enhanced, spirits may materialize, and perhaps a cosmic bridge or smoke tunnel appears, allowing the shaman to ascend to the heavens.

Today such consciousness-altering plants tend to be classified as illegal. While they can be toxic, they are not poisonous unless abused by those who do not respect their powers. Among some indigenous peoples sacred plants were used only by the shaman or medicine man for the specific purpose of obtaining knowledge from the spirit world about healing a patient or for the welfare of the whole community.

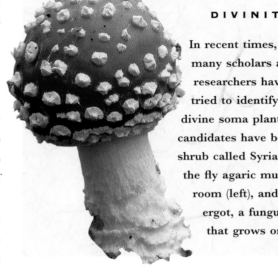

DIVINITY

In recent times, many scholars and researchers have tried to identify the divine soma plant. Top candidates have been a shrub called Syrian rue, the fly agaric mushroom (left), and ergot, a fungus that grows on rye.

Those plants traditionally used by the shaman or medicine man to access sacred healing knowledge include angel's trumpet (*p. 118*) in Hawaii, henbane in Europe (*p. 128*) and morning glory (*p. 131*) in Mexico. Flowers of these plants have been made into flower essences that do not contain any trace of chemicals, only the flower's energy, so they can be used quite safely. In Central and South America a wealth of other psychoactive plants are used in rituals and ceremonies that cannot be recommended because they are potentially poisonous (and illegal), but their place among the plant spirit medicines cannot be overlooked.

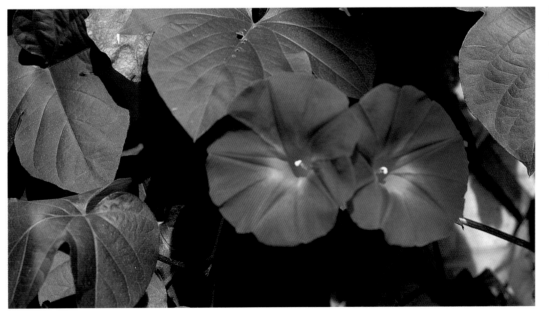

LEFT *Morning Glory. Many toxic plants induce hallucinations. While these might be dangerous, they are nevertheless part of the world of plant spirits.*

Banisteriopsis caapi – AYAHUASCA

A most sacred jungle vine used more than 3,000 years by the people living in the Andes and Amazonian jungle. It is regarded as a powerful healing medicine. Ayahuasca translates as "vine of the soul." The shaman or medicine man is the keeper of ayahuasca's secrets. One type of ayahuasca allows the shaman to contact the spirits of animals who bring their special energy medicine to those in need of healing. Another is revered as a teacher of medicine. Traditionally the bark is brewed to make a beverage sipped by the shaman during a sacred ceremony. After taking ayahuasca, the shaman may develop an ability to see into the physical body to diagnose disease. When given to the patient, ayahuasca appears to heal by taking the person on a spiritual journey of self-discovery. It awakens intuition, imagination, the ability to see and face the truth about oneself and one's life. The visionary qualities of ayahuasca are due to harmala alkaloids, once known as "telepathine," because of their apparent ability to stimulate extrasensory perception. People who use ayahuasca believe it releases negative vibrations or energy patterns resulting from destructive thought processes and trauma that are held in the body. Recent research shows ayahuasca does possess regenerative properties and helps to repair the overloaded neurones in the brain.

Lophophora williamsii – PEYOTE

The famous peyote cactus, whose name derives from the Aztec "peyotl," is primarily associated with the Huichol Indians of the Sierra Madre in Mexico. Traditionally, the shaman, who is in contact with the peyote god, Tatewari, leads a pilgrimage covering many miles to the desert of San Luis Potosi, known as "Wirikuta," where peyote grows. The cactus is collected, broken into small pieces or mashed and mixed with water, then shared among the participants. The Huichols identify the peyote with the sacred deer who takes them to the upper levels of the cosmos and is a spirit helper who can be called upon during healing ceremonies. Peyote contains around 30 psychoactive agents, the main one being mescaline. Users experience vividly colored images, shimmering auras around objects, a feeling of weightlessness, and unusual sensory changes. It is said that peyote enables one to foresee and predict future events.

Trichocereus pachanol – SAN PEDRO CACTUS

The ritual use of San Pedro, one of South America's most ancient magical plants, dates back at least 3,000 years. The shamans of tribes living in Peru and Bolivia drink a beverage made from the sap of the cactus as a means of contacting spirits, treating illness, and predicting future events. Like peyote, San Pedro contains mescaline, which evokes a state of dreamy lethargy that later gives way to lucid mental images. The shaman or "curandero" claims the San Pedro enables his spirit to rise or descend into the supernatural realms. By stimulating the sixth sense, it allows the shaman to "see" into the patient's psyche and discover the source of their unhappiness and ill-health.

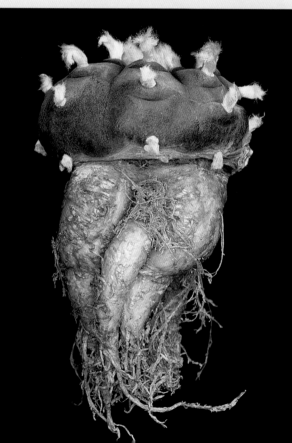

LEFT *The peyote brings enlightenment, attuning the user with the forces of nature and facilitating communication with plant and animal spirits.*

North America

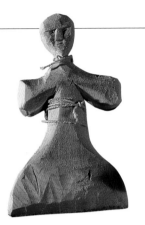

Fᴏʀ ʜᴜɴᴅʀᴇᴅs ᴏꜰ *years before the arrival of European settlers, the enormous North American continent was inhabited by peoples who knew it as Turtle Island. These Native Americans endeavored to live in harmony with the world of nature and everything in it.*

ABOVE *Native Americans have left behind many symbols of their religious beliefs.*

The Native Americans regard themselves as caretakers or keepers of the land, responsible for safeguarding its fertility. They have always seen themselves as belonging to the natural world, and as inhabitants of Turtle Island felt it was their duty not to act in a way that would disturb the balance that existed in nature. The island was their home and they regarded it as sacred.

LEGENDS

Native American legends tell of Gentle Giants who once walked upon the earth in times when all was peace and harmony. These giants were reputedly a highly spiritual people who believed the Great Spirit, *Gitchi Manitou*, was present in all things. It is said that they conversed freely with the nature spirits of animals, flowers, the wind, water, and thunder. They could also utilize these energies for healing purposes. In Native American societies today, the ability to sense the subtle energies lives on in their shamans, priests, and medicine men and women.

CEREMONIES

Each tribe has its own word that signifies the sacred center, the divine source from which all things have

ABOVE *Ceremonies in honour of Gitchi Manitou are an important part of Native American ritual life.*
RIGHT *There are many legends of giants and spiritual beings in North American history.*

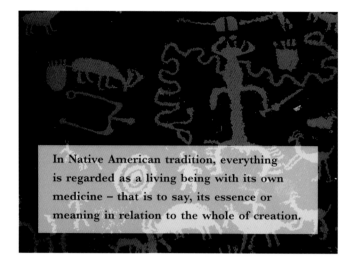

In Native American tradition, everything is regarded as a living being with its own medicine – that is to say, its essence or meaning in relation to the whole of creation.

come. The Sioux word is "wakan," the Ojiwa "manido," the Omaha "wakanda" and the Mandan "ho'pinis."

Sacred ceremonies are performed to ensure the well-being of the whole community. The sacred pipe ceremony and medicine wheel act as a means of periodically renewing the connection with all that is sacred in nature. Forgetting one's place in the web of life is felt to lead to illness and disharmony.

Sage, a most sacred plant, is used as a smudging tool during such ceremonies to clear away any negative energies, sometimes in combination with wormwood, sweetgrass, or cedar. Sage is also employed in the sweat lodge ceremony, an ancient purifying and healing ritual that symbolizes a leaving behind of old habits and a rebirth of the spirit. It signifies a step in spiritual evolution.

HEALING

To the Native Americans, sickness is associated with disease of the spirit, and healing aims to promote a sense of spiritual well-being as well as relieving any emotional, mental, and physical ills. Some tribes believe that spirits inspire the healer to know which curative plants to use, others that a plant is protected by the spirit that has endowed it with medicinal properties. Offerings, usually of the sacred plant tobacco, are often left to these spirits when the healing plant is picked. Typical native plants used as spirit medicines include osha (*p.136*), purple cone flower (*p.120*), angelica (*p.100*) and evening primrose (*p.148*).

ABOVE *Sacred gifts were left to the plant spirit when the plant was picked.*

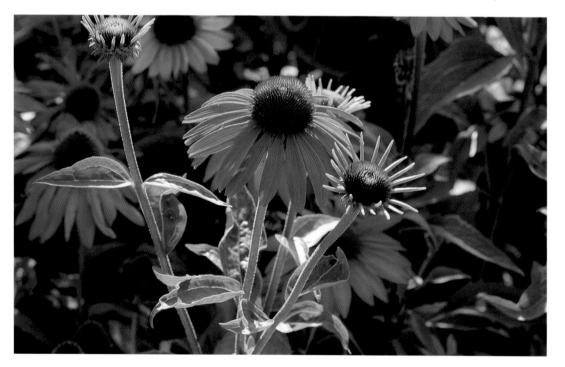

RIGHT *The purple cone flower was used in spirit medicines by Native Americans.*

Central and South America

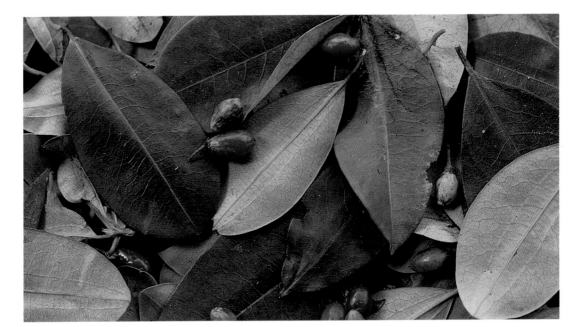

THIS VAST AND *colorful continent is home to many magical plants and flowers, possessing both healing and visionary qualities. The use of* plant spirit medicines by the people of Central and South America is legendary and can be traced back to the earliest times.

ABOVE *Quetzalcoatl, the Toltec and Aztec god.*

RIGHT *The coca plant is a typical product of South America.*

The Aztecs who once dominated Central America had a sophisticated knowledge of healing plants. They saw godlike qualities in plants such as maize and sunflower, used visionary plants such as peyote and morning glory as divine remedies for healing purposes, and employed many others as medicines. When the Spanish conquered Mexico in the sixteenth century they discovered around 1,200 plants in the Aztec pharmacopoeia.

LEGENDS

These people attributed their knowledge and belief systems to a legendary god-king named Quetzalcoatl who reputedly lived in a golden age, came to Mexico from a far-off land, and achieved immortality through spiritual purification. This god was also worshiped by the Maya of the Yuctan, Chiaptas,

and Guatemala whose descendants are scattered throughout Central America.

The Mayan medicine men are still masters of plant spirit medicine, using visionary plants to connect with the nature spirits who in turn provide visions of other healing plants. The sacred smoke of copal is used as a diagnostic tool, enabling the shamans to see disharmony in the subtle energies of the person they are treating.

SOUTH AMERICA

From the Amazonian rainforests to the mountainous regions of Peru, we find people with a reverence for nature and who use their healing plants in a sacred way.

Nestling between three sacred Andean mountain peaks, about 12,000ft./3,600m above sea level, is Machu Picchu.

The Incas performed rituals and ceremonies at this site using the sacred coca plant, as did an earlier people about whom little is known but who, like the Inca high priests, may have been keepers of the ancient mystical traditions.

The secret teachings of the Incas parallel the spiritual beliefs of the Q'ueros, a Quechua-speaking people living today in remote mountain villages above the holy city of Cuzco. The Q'ueros believe that everything is imbued with spirit. Like many other people living throughout South America, they regard the Earth Mother, or Pachamama, as the true spiritual mother who holds the secrets of the universe. They refer to the earth energies or nature spirits as apus, who are the guardians of Pachamama. All the skills that the Q'ueros priests, or paqos, learn are to do with the harmonious interplay of energies. The shaman's gift is the ability to heal his people's relationship with the cosmic forces in ways that bring harmony and balance into their lives. The "despacho" ceremony is a traditional way of honoring Pachamama and preserving harmonious relationships with the energies. The "kurak" (priest shaman) lays his ceremonial tools or mantas before him, draws a fistful of coca leaves from his pouch, and utters a prayer to sacred coca before letting them fall over the mantas. Sharing the coca leaves is an important sacred act of spiritual and energetic bonding.

RIGHT *A Quechua woman from Peru, whose beliefs echo those of the Incas.*

BELOW *The lost magical city of the Incas, Machu Picchu, in Peru.*

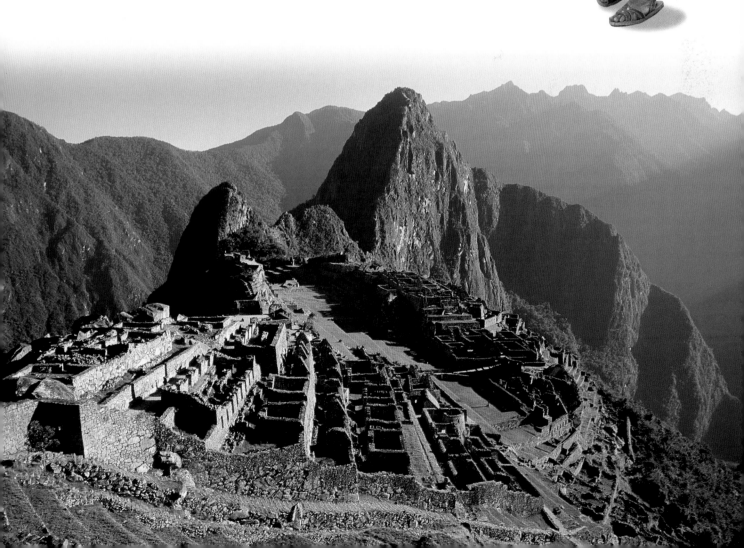

Europe and Scandinavia

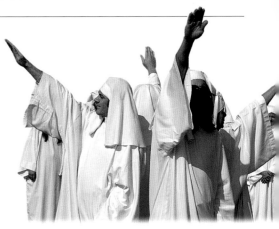

I N ANCIENT TIMES, *the people of Europe and Scandinavia felt that nature was sacred. They practiced an earth-orientated religion that honored the mother goddess and her nature spirits. Tree worship was widespread and certain trees such as oak, ash, elder, and hawthorn were seen as having particularly magical properties.*

ABOVE *The Druid religion in Western Europe dates back many centuries.*

A mystical people known as the Druids are thought to have been guardians of this sacred lore and wisdom. The ancient Druids left no written clues as to their beliefs and traditions, but the invading Romans recorded them as being skilled in the art of magic, astrology, healing, music, and poetry. They worshiped in sacred groves, venerated the oak above all trees, and saw mistletoe growing on this tree as evidence of a divine presence.

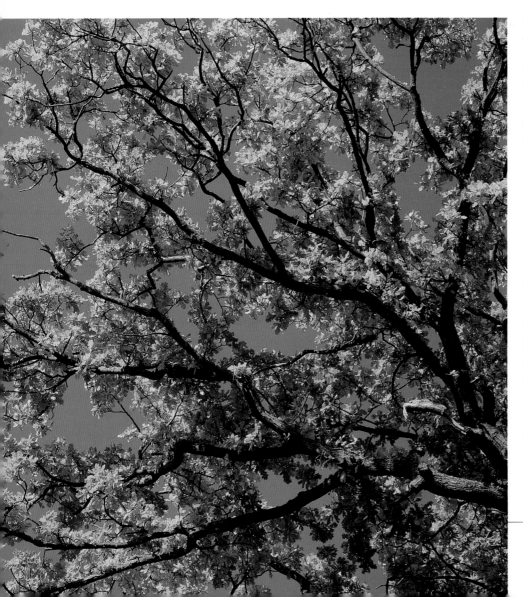

CEREMONIES

With the advent of Christianity, ceremonies for honoring nature such as May day, the winter and summer solstices, and gathering the harvest, were deemed pagan. But so deeply ingrained was the earth religion in European culture that these were not forgotten. They literally became absorbed into the Christian calendar under different guises.

The Church was also suspicious of the spiritual element of healing with plants and herbs. It is possible that European medicine men, or more commonly women, took perception-enhancing plants such as henbane in a sacred or magical way, which gave rise to the concept of

LEFT *The turning of the seasons is marked by many festivals in the Christian calendar.*

witchcraft. But knowledge of medicinal plants was not extinguished. It was studied by the monks and kept alive in the seclusion and comparative safety of their cloisters. The notion of nature spirits also survived, and these divine entities resurfaced in the guise of the fairies, pixies, elves, and sprites described in traditional European folklore and fairytales.

SCANDINAVIA

Tales of Thor, the god of thunder, and descriptions of Yggdrasil, or the tree of life, in Norse mythology, hint of a once deeply rooted belief amongst Scandinavians in the divine powers of nature.

Not so long ago, Laplanders living within the Arctic Circle practiced a true form of shamanism. With his staff of life, swirling cloak of animal skins, and magic drum, the Lapp holy man, or shaman, must have been an imposing figure. As well as chanting and drumming himself into a trance-like state, the Lapp shaman also knew how to prepare the "magical" or hallucinogenic fly agaric mushroom (*Amanita muscaria*). It is said his spirit took the form of an animal and

THE FLY AGARIC MUSHROOM

The fly agaric mushroom played an important role in the Lapp's semidomestication of the reindeer. These creatures are the only animals known to intoxicate themselves voluntarily with fly agaric. The mushrooms make them docile and manageable. The popular image of Santa Claus and his flying reindeer appears to be an interpretation of the shaman's journey. Santa's costume is reminiscent of the mushroom, which is bright red with white spots.

flew to other realms to communicate with the spirits of nature. Many of the plants traditionally used as spirit medicines in this region are classified as adaptogens. In other words they possess qualities that help the body to adapt to stress and so survive in the harsh climatic conditions. They include Nordic ginseng or kvanna (see *Panax*), acantho root or cari-oga as it is known in Sweden, and arctic root (see *Angelica*), a Nordic form of angelica.

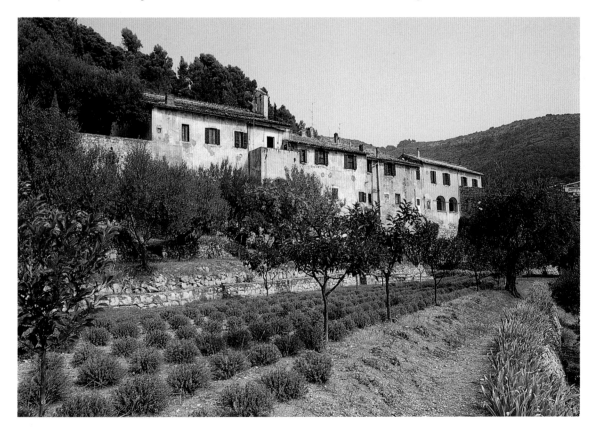

LEFT *A monastery near Tivoli, Italy. Early Christian monks studied the medicinal qualities of plants.*

The Mediterranean and the Middle East

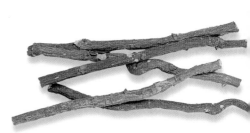

ABOVE *Trees and bark have always been held sacred in the Middle East.*

THIS REGION OF *the world is known as the cradle of civilization. Many centuries ago its people developed a wealth of religious concepts and spiritual ideals, including a belief in the sacredness of trees, plants, and flowers.*

An image of the sacred tree was used by Akkadians dwelling in the Sumerian city of Eridu on the shores of the Persian Gulf between 4000 and 3000 B.C.E. It takes the form of a date palm, pomegranate, cypress or vine, suggesting all these plants were deified. The symbol was associated with Ishtar, the divine mother goddess.

The famous Code of Hammurabi written by the Babylonian king (1792–1750 B.C.E.) contains references to healing plants including henbane, licorice, mint, hemp (cannabis), and opium poppy, known as the plant of joy. The Greek historian Herodotus tells us that in Babylon's heyday 57,320lb./26,000kg of frankincense was burned on the golden altars in religious ceremonies, further evidence that these people sought contact with the sacred.

ABOVE *Ancient Egyptian priests used aromatic plants to encourage spiritual contemplation in temples.*

ANCIENT EGYPT

The power of the ancient Egyptian healer-physicians is legendary. According to the Homer their skills in medicine exceeded those of any others. Many trees, plants, and flowers were seen to possess divine or godlike qualities.

The Pharaoh, high priests, and temple initiates were preoccupied with spiritual perfection as a means of preparing the soul to take its place among the stars in the afterlife. Frankincense, myrrh, and other aromatic plants were burned in temples to encourage spiritual contemplation. Each god was associated with a particular plant or its fragrance.

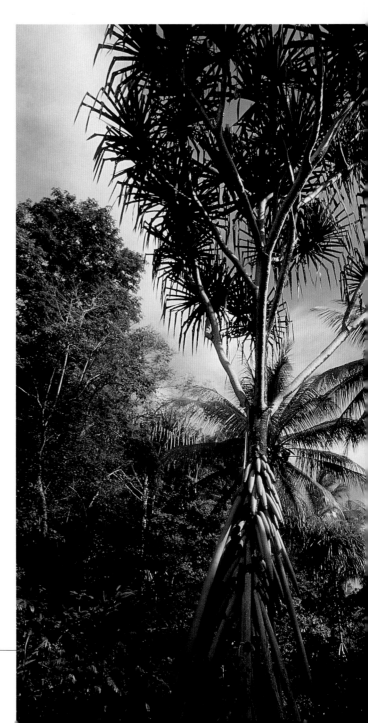

On auspicious days, statues of Isis would be anointed with sweet-smelling artemisia and those of Osiris with marjoram. Essential oils and other plant preparations were used as medicines and beauty treatments. A perfect spirit deserved a beautiful body. The ancient Egyptians also invented a language of flowers and conveyed messages with bouquets rather than letters.

ANCIENT GREECE

Greeks living in classical times marveled at Egyptian culture but were more influenced by the traditions of the Minoans living in Crete. On this Mediterranean isle dwelt an advanced sea-faring people (they invented writing) who revered nature and worshiped Mother Earth.

In early times the Greek gods and goddesses inhabited plants and trees. Zeus took the form of the oak; laurel was sacred to Apollo; and Artemis – an independent divinity closely related to wood nymphs and wild vegetation – was envisaged as the cedar, laurel, and myrtle. Wreaths and branches also retained a vestige of the power attributed to the spirit of the trees. The use of blossoms and leaves was an expression of religious emotion. They also realized the healing potential of plants, and esteemed Greek scholars such as Hippocrates, Aristotle, Theophrastus, and Dioscorides wrote treatises and compiled pharmacopoeias. These provided the basis for the great European herbals, which were among the first books to be published following the invention of the printing press.

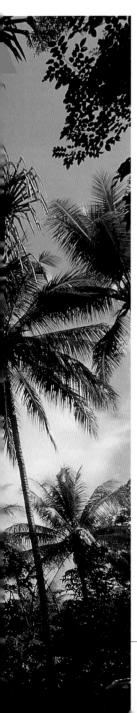

LEFT *The Mediterranean climate is ideal for growing many plants with sweet-smelling, oily flowers and leaves, useful for medicine and beauty treatments.*

THE BOOK OF THOTH

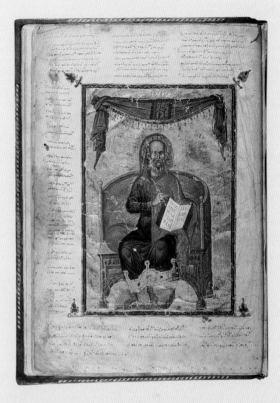

According to Egyptian mythology, all cures were revealed by the gods and interpreted by Thoth, a mortal who achieved immortality through self-purification. The Book of Thoth reputedly contained his teachings on astronomy, astrology, medicine, philosophy, and religion.

LEFT *The ancient Greeks wore blossoms and leaves into wreaths, which retained some of the power of the spirit of the tree.*

Africa

SCATTERED THROUGHOUT AFRICA *are many tribes, such as the Masai and Kikuyu, whose traditions and belief systems are deeply rooted in the past. Vestiges of the earliest phase of magical and religious thinking, known as animism, linger on.*

Africa is a country in which spirits or souls are thought to inhabit the hills, trees, rocks, streams, and oceans although they are not necessarily tied to a particular place. These spirits are thought to exert a strong influence over the welfare of humankind, and for this reason they are treated with great respect.

Every village along the Guinea coast has its own sacred tree that is endowed with special powers. The iroko (African oak), silk-cotton, baobab, acacia, mahogany, and palm trees are the most revered species, although several shrubs are also considered sacred.

Myths tell how men and women descended to earth from the branches of a huge mythical loko, the Dahomey word for iroko. Some still think the souls of those about to be born live in trees or thickets of bamboo. Women often pray to the spirits of trees to send them children. Prayers and gifts are offered to the sacred trees in times of sickness.

WITCH DOCTORS

In most traditional African cultures there exists a belief that disease is caused by malevolent spirits, often associated with the souls of ancestors, which may be offended in various ways. Disease is kept at bay by observing taboos, wearing amulets, giving offerings to the spirits, or by ritual dancing. If a person falls sick his or her spiritual welfare is called into question.

RIGHT *Masai tribespeople from Kenya, East Africa, still adhere to traditional ways and beliefs in a spirit world.*

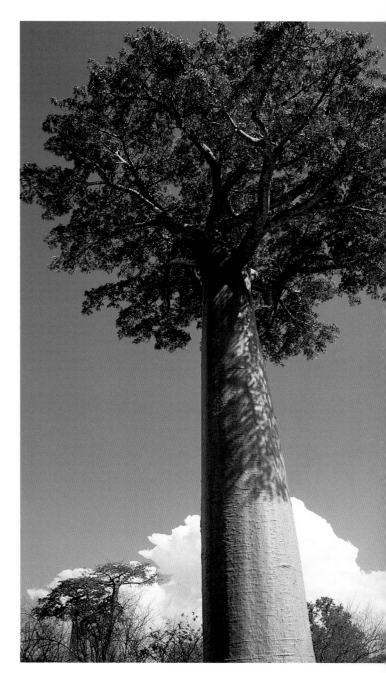

RIGHT *The baobab or "monkey-bread" tree. Throughout Africa, the roots, bark, and leaves of many trees are believed to have healing powers.*

Healers are both medicine men and priests, attending to all aspects of the people's well-being. The tribal witch doctors believe there are unseen powers, secrets that can be tapped and laws set in motion by the knowledgeable. A good doctor possesses such skills and is also well acquainted with the healing powers of the roots, barks, leaves, and stems of local flora. Herbs or healing plants are essential ingredients to most medicines, which are said to house a spiritual being, power, or breath of life. To evoke its true healing potential, the medicine is activated by the magical charms and chants of the doctor. For a medicine to be effective it must please the patient's soul, for one of the commonest causes of sickness is a troubled soul.

In southern Ethiopia live a people known as the Borana whose culture is at least 3,000 years old and who consider themselves to be among the most spiritually evolved people on earth. The spiritual welfare of the tribe lies in the hands of high priests called qaalus, and within the small commu-

SACRED PLANTS

The most sacred plant in West Africa is the shrub called iboga (*Tabernanthe iboga*) revered for the visionary states it induces. The Fang tribe of Gabon still use it ritually in coming-of-age ceremonies to initiate their young people into connecting with the ancestor spirits. Among the most sacred plants of the Australian Aborigines are the various species of native fuchsia, or emu bush, 18 of which are used medicinally. The Alyawarra of Central Australia use seven for colds, flu, headaches, chest pains, fever, diarrhea, and wounds, among other ailments.

nity there are also "daballe," specially gifted people who are considered to be mediators between humans and the supreme god, Waq. The daballe are psychics, mystics, astronomers, and expert herbalists who are guided in all aspects of life, including their healing work, by nature spirits, the ancestors, and the stars. For, like the Dogon in West Africa, these people believe their ancestors originally came from the stars and that we are part of a vast interconnected web of life.

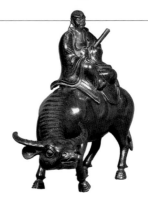

India, the Himalayas, and Tibet

T HE HIMALAYAS HAVE *a magical quality that has long attracted those seeking divine inspiration and enlightenment, including Lao Tzu, the founder of Taoism. Reaching through the clouds to the heavens, the mountains symbolize the peak of consciousness.*

ABOVE *India and Tibet have long been regarded as the place where the secrets of spiritual enlightenment might be revealed.*

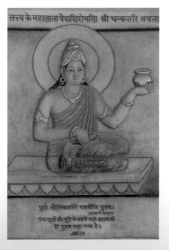

The wisdom of the yogis was passed on by word of mouth through the centuries before being written down in the Vedas or Books of Knowledge. Their philosophies form the basis of the Hindu religion and a form of natural medicine known as Ayurveda. Healing embraced the well-being of mind, body, and spirit, with plants and flowers playing an essential role in promoting harmony and balance. Hinduism sees divinity as a natural part of the world, not something separate; it exists in

rocks and rivers, mountains and caves, plants and trees. The Vedas describe certain plant and tree species as incarnations or symbols of deities and these feature in a number of religious ceremonies, offerings, and prayers.

Plants with exquisite perfumes such as jasmine and sandalwood, are highly revered

LEFT *The philosophy of the yogis encompasses well-being of the body, mind, and spirit.*

BELOW *Hinduism and Buddhism have their roots in the Himalayas.*

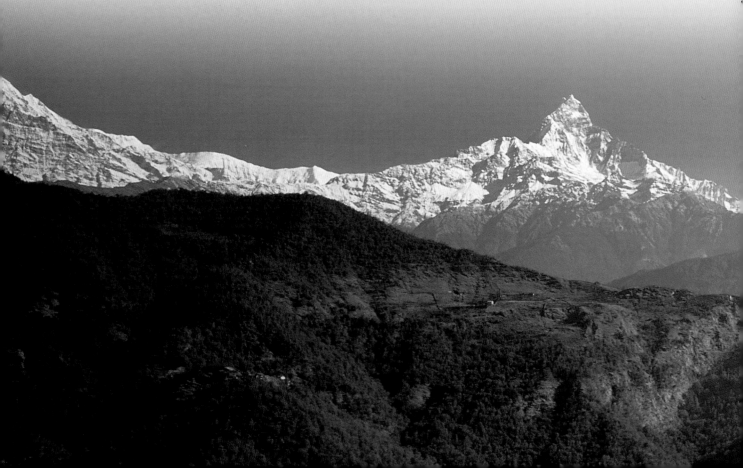

for they evoke pleasure, whose pursuit is a part of Indian spiritual philosophy. In Ayurvedic medicine, plant oils are massaged into the skin to evoke feelings of bliss, while essential oils and herbal teas are prescribed according to your personality and mind-body type. The Vedas reveal an extensive knowledge of healing plants, while the Charaka Somhita, a later Indian herbal, mentions more than 500 plant remedies (richer than the Egyptian pharmacopoeias), many of which were adopted in Egypt, then Greece, and finally found their way into European folk medicine.

THE BIRTH OF BUDDHISM

India is also the birthplace of Buddhism, a spiritual philosophy that evolved during the fifth century B.C.E. Motivated by the quest to attain long-lasting contentment and inner peace through mental, spiritual, and moral development, a young prince named Siddhartha Gautama took up the life of a wandering ascetic in northern India. Enlightenment eventually came to him sitting under the Bodhi, or Bo Tree, which is considered in Buddhism to be the oldest and most holy tree in the world. In Tibet, Buddhism exists in harmony with an ancient shamanic view of the world.

THE LOTUS

The most sacred flower in India has always been the lotus. In Hindu mythology, Brahma, the supreme deity, emerged from its unfurling petals. Its white color denotes purity, while the unfolding action of its petals symbolizes the process of becoming. It is also India's national flower.

The shaman of the Bon religion sees illness arising from an energy imbalance that humans create between themselves and all existence when they upset the spirits of nature. Healing involves contacting the nye, or tree spirits, and the sadag, or earth spirits of the mountains, rivers, plants, clouds, and sky, to reestablish harmonious relationships with them. Nangshen are purification rituals designed to liberate any negative energy and appease the nature spirits with offerings. The shaman then summons powerful energy from all corners of the universe, condenses it into syllables, and introduces them through the crown chakra to reinforce the person's life force, or chilu, which keeps mind, body, and soul together.

Siberia and the Far East

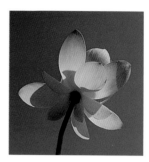

S HAMAN IS A *Russian word originally used to denote the medicine people of certain Siberian tribes. The native Siberians, living in the vast region stretching from the Urals in the west to the Altai mountains in the south and the Arctic Ocean in the north, still practice shamanism and believe everything that exists has a spirit.*

ABOVE *The lotus is the most sacred flower of the Far East, holding the wisdom of the world.*

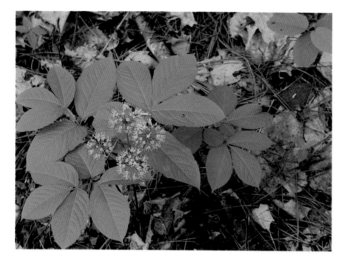

CHINA AND JAPAN

The Immortals of the Mountains were an early Chinese people who thought mountain mist contained potent concentrations of qi, or chi, the vital essence of life. In their quest for immortality, they searched for plants and herbs with powers to nurture, strengthen, and prolong life.

LEFT *The Altai people searched for plants they believed could prolong life.*

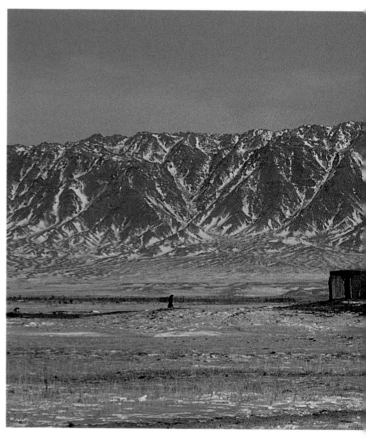

The Altai people call their healer-priests kams, meaning messengers between the human and spirit worlds. Kams are thought to possess magical powers and look after the spiritual welfare of the community as well as each individual. The Altai talk of evil spirits, too, that drain vital energy.

The kams use many of the mountain plants in a sacred way for healing. Roots are often burned and inhaled, flowers and leaves made into tinctures, and others are simply carried. The matagora or golden root is an acclaimed elixir of life and was used by hunters to enhance perception, bringing visions and allowing them to see auras. Hemp (cannabis) leaves may have been smoked for this purpose whilst its seeds are traditionally ground to make a nutritious butter. Hemp oil is now recognised as one of nature's best sources of essential fatty acids and has remarkable healing properties. The Altai see the goal of spiritual development as realizing we each have a celestial being in our heart. Becoming one with this person opens the door to immortality.

Vestiges of their beliefs and traditions appear in Taoism, a philosophy of life taught by Lao Tzu, who urged people to model their behavior on the Tao or "way of nature." Taoism sees the universe as a living organism that is infused and permeated with an energy or life force that moves through all things (see page 27). Following the Tao brings an abundance of free-flowing qi, which in turn holds the key to happiness and perfect health. Herbs and healing plants are part of a philosophy that nurtures spiritual growth and the benefits it bestows. Early Taoists felt their spiritual destination to be "a mythical island of the Eastern Sea where there existed a herb with the power to bestow immortality."

The indigenous religion of Japan is Shinto, meaning the Way of Kami (or way of the gods). An abiding reverence toward nature stems from a belief that spirit beings or gods occupy and govern the natural world. Japanese mythology tells of holy sakaki trees growing on the Mountain of Heaven and of a herb of immortality that can be gathered from the Island of Eternal Youth.

Ritual purification, or oharai, is still performed by a priest who waves a sacred sakaki (prosperity tree) over the person's head. Worshipers believe the oharai removes accumulated pollution and restores internal bodily equilibrium as well as harmonious relationships with the outer world.

ABOVE *Evidence of a shaman's presence in the mountains of Mongolia.*

BELOW *The Altai Mountains in China are home to many plants used for healing.*

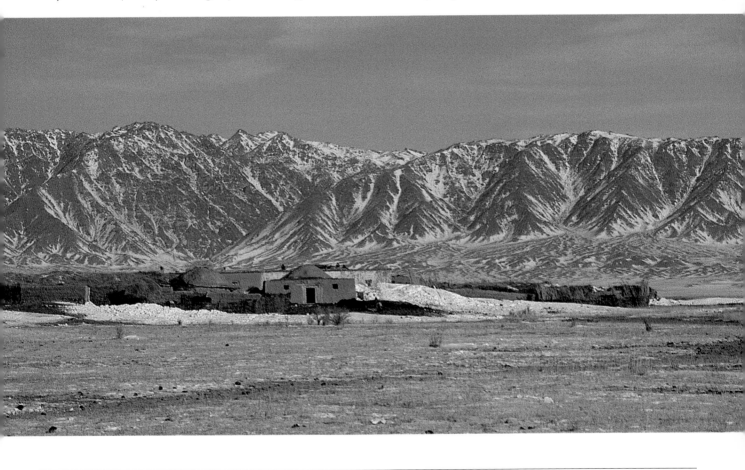

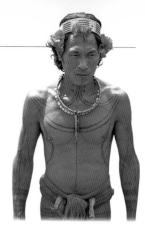

Indonesia, the Pacific Islands, and Australia

A BELIEF IN THE *sacredness of nature is found among indigenous people living on islands throughout the South Pacific. Ancestral traditions play an important role in the healing practices used today.*

ABOVE *The shaman is able to prescribe the perfect plant remedy by sensing sickness in others.*

Diverse cultures and religious beliefs mingle throughout Indonesia, yet many native islanders have faith in the powers of the medicine man who performs the same sort of feats and functions as shamans found elsewhere in the world. There are healers who claim to sense the vibrations emitted by plants and herbs. Typically he or she enters a state of meditation or mindfulness to enhance sensitivity to the vibrational qualities of a plant. At the same time, he senses sickness or energetic disharmony in the body, which enables him to prescribe the perfect plant remedy.

HAWAII AND THE PACIFIC ISLANDS

Around 2,000 years ago, sea-faring people from Pacific islands made their home among the string of volcanic islands forming the Hawaiian archipelago. These Polynesians brought many of their favorite plants including the kukui, hau, and milo trees and grew ti plants around their houses and temples to ward off evil spirits.

Native Hawaiians believe in a creative life force, known as mana, necessary for the growth of all life forms. In Hawaii, exotic flowers in vibrant hues are threaded together to form the traditional headbands, or leis, and garlands worn during sacred ceremonies to honor their deities and welcome guests onto the islands.

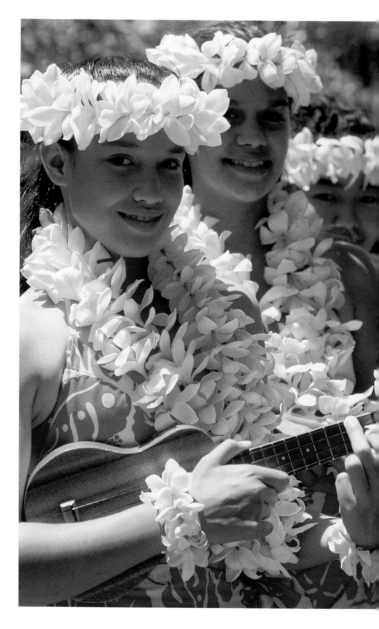

RIGHT *Hawaiian garlands honor deities during ceremonies.*

The Hawaiians show great care, or kokua, for their plants and give them names that reflect an appreciation of each one's characteristics. They believe divine beings known as aumakua act as guardians to plants. Those used in healing are treated with great reverence and respect. To the South Sea Islanders of Oceania kava kava (*Piper methysticum*) is sacred and features in many aspects of their culture. An intoxicating brew is drunk during rituals and ceremonies whilst a milder version is offered to welcome guests. Kava is now recognized for its ability to instil calm and peacefulness, which may explain why these people have been dubbed the happiest in the world!

AUSTRALIA

The current beliefs and traditions of the native Aborigines are rooted in their ancestry. The Nyoongah people of South West Australia say that flowers remind them of how life was restored, for they carry the colors of the Creator Spirit or Rainbow Snake who pierced the Ice allowing Sun Woman to warm the earth.

LEFT A sacred ceremonial brew of kava offers a sense of calm and peace.

The dreamtime is their mythical past when the gods brought the world into being and the ancestors sang the world alive. Maintaining contact with the ancestors is essential to Aborigines, and at traditional ceremonies the elders chant and dance themselves into a trance in which they are able to step into the dreamtime. The songs they sing today are said to be those the ancestors sang in the distant past.

Their healing knowledge and traditions also spring from the dreamtime. The Nyoongah live surrounded by blossoming wild flowers to which they attribute healing properties. The mobarn or wadinyoongahri are the tribal healers who conduct a healing ceremony whereby a person becomes immersed in the floral energy. They place a layer of hot coals in a pit of earth, sprinkle it with water and flowers, and cover it with a layer of kangaroo skin, creating a sauna. The flowers are thought to renew the spirit. The frightened gain courage, the angry find peace, and the sick become well.

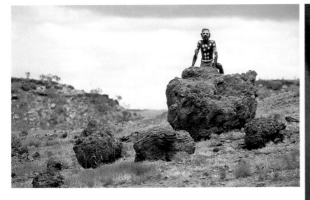

ABOVE Australian Aborigines have connections with the spirit world derived from the teachings of their ancestors.

RIGHT Among the most sacred plants of the Australian Aborigines are the various species of native fuchsia or emu bush, eighteen of which are used medicinally. The fringed lily twiner builds a gracious, loving nature.

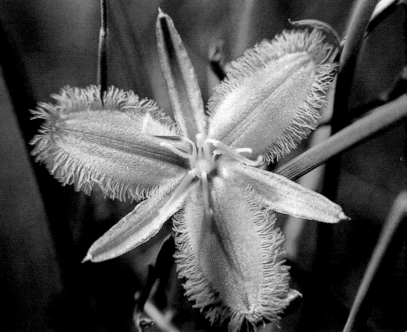

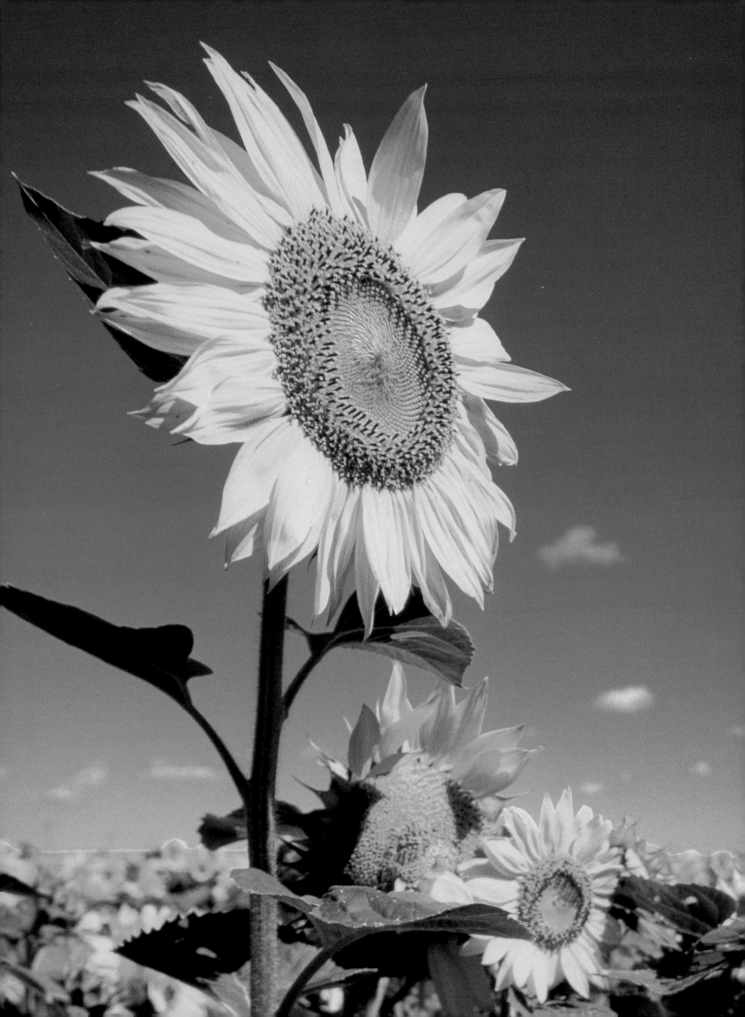

FLOWER AND PLANT ENCYCLOPEDIA

Yarrow

LATIN NAME: *Achillea millefolium*
FAMILY: *Compositae*

"My gift is to protect with a shield of light, revitalizing and repairing the aura."

Yarrow is one of the oldest healing plants. Once a first-aid herb for warriors, it has wonderful powers for remedying any harm or injury to the physical and energetic bodies.

SPIRIT AND SYMBOLISM

Some 60,000 years ago, Neanderthal people buried their dead with flowers and medicinal plants, including yarrow. This was discovered by Ralph Solecki while excavating a pre-historic site in Shanidar, once in the northern province of Mesopotamia. People living in this region still use yarrow as an important healing herb. An unassuming plant with feather-like leaves and bouquets of white florets, yarrow is a master healer capable of repairing physical wounds and damage to the aura.

Yarrow was greatly valued by ancient Greeks. They named it after the heroic warrior Achilles, who is credited

Yarrow was originally discovered in Northern Iraq. It can now also be found in Greece, North America, and North Europe.

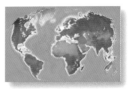

with being the first person to use its mysterious healing flowers on himself and his soldiers when treating wounds suffered on the battlefield.

Yarrow is also used as a visionary herb that enhances the ability to see beyond the realms of reality, providing it is cut on the night of a full moon. Ayurvedics use the herb as a "heal-all" because it has so many uses. Yarrow stalks are used as divining tools in the ancient Chinese oracle, the *I Ching*.

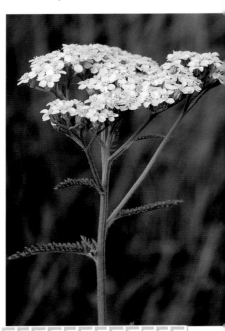

RIGHT *To get the yarrow plant at its best, gather it in early summer.*

PLANT SPIRIT MEDICINES

An infusion of yarrow flowers has antiseptic and astringent qualities for cleansing

LEFT *Yarrow can help those who spend a lot of time in front of the computer.*

wounds, inhibiting inflammation, and promoting healing. Yarrow can also balance emotional upsets. In homeopathy, *Achillea millefolium* is indicated for nosebleeds, profuse menstrual bleeding, hemorrhages, and a

constant high temperature.

As a flower essence, yarrow strengthens the aura and brings protection from energetic environmental hazards, such as electromagnetic radiation from computers and fluorescent lights.

Garlic

LATIN NAME: *Allium sativum*

FAMILY: *Alliaceae*

"My pungent aroma purifies and protects the mind and body."

With its unmistakable scent, this plant is renowned the world over for its health-enhancing properties. The spirit of garlic is like a lifesaver who safeguards and protects those in his care.

SPIRIT AND SYMBOLISM

From its oval leaves and bulbs to its white starry flowers, the whole plant radiates the distinctive garlicky scent.

Garlic's purifying and protective spirit has been recognized for centuries. It is one of the oldest known medicinal plants; a remedy using garlic was found on a Sumerian clay tablet which dated back to 3000 B.C.E. The ancient Egyptians used garlic to stave off epidemic and it was given to Hebrew slaves during the building of the pyramids to preserve good health. Garlic was also thought to ward off evil spirits, and cloves of it were discovered in the tomb of Tutankhamun and the sacred animal temple at Saqqara. In Eastern European folklore, garlic is renowned for warding off vampires, while in England to dream of garlic symbolizes good luck.

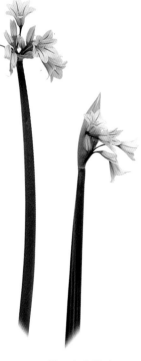

ABOVE *Plant individual cloves in the fall to grow your own garlic.*

LEFT *Garlic cloves can be chewed, cooked, powdered, or taken as an infusion, decoction, or tea.*

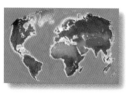

PLANT SPIRIT MEDICINES

Garlic's antiseptic and antibiotic powers are legendary. Eaten regularly, fresh garlic prevents colds and flu, but if you succumb it can help to loosen mucus and clear coughs. A potent lung cleanser, garlic can help asthma and hay fever. Added to food or taken as an oil, garlic boosts the circulation, decreases blood clotting factors, and lowers blood pressure, so protecting the heart from disease.

Aged garlic helps maintain healthy reproductive organs in both sexes and protects against cancer, a benefit recognized by Hippocrates in the fourth century B.C. Giving garlic to children helps to ward off threadworms.

As a flower essence, garlic helps those who are fearful, weak, and easily influenced, which makes them vulnerable to all kinds of ills. It bolsters psychological resistance and boosts spiritual strength.

ABOVE *Garlic can help ease childhood coughs and colds.*

Aloe Vera

LATIN NAME: *Aloe communis*

FAMILY: *Aloeaceae*

"I hold the power to repair and replenish the aura."

Native Americans call the leaves of aloe vera "wands of heaven" because of their amazing healing powers. Growing in arid desert regions, aloe vera is a cactus-like plant blessed with the ability to repair damage caused by the harshest elements of life, promoting the healing of wounds and burns.

SPIRIT AND SYMBOLISM

Distinguished by its vivid, yellow spiked blooms and succulent leaves filled with a sap that soothes and heals all kinds of damage, the spirit of aloe is resilient and self-reliant. According to popular legend, aloes were present in the Garden of Eden. The therapeutic use of aloe juice dates back at least 3,500 years and ancient records suggest that the renowned Egyptian beauty Cleopatra bathed in aloe vera as well as asses' milk. For centuries, the Sultan of Socotra had a strict monopoly on aloe and it is said that Alexander the Great conquered the island and seized this plant praised by the early Greek physician Dioscorides for its ability to soothe burns and stomach ulcers.

ABOVE Soothing sap is extracted from the leaves of the aloe vera.

ORIGIN

A native of eastern and southern Africa, wild aloe vera grows in tropical countries. It is also cultivated worldwide.

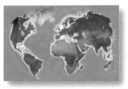

PLANT SPIRIT MEDICINES

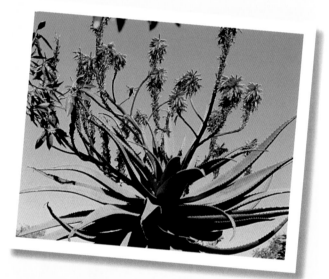

ABOVE *Tenacious aloe vera grows to amazing heights even in the harshest of conditions.*

Pure aloe vera gel is rich in vitamins C, B1, B2, and B6, calcium and potassium salts, active enzymes, natural sugars, and some 18 different amino acids. Applied to the skin, aloe soothes burns, moisturizes, and speeds the regeneration of healthy new cells, making it an excellent ingredient for treating sunburned skin. It is also helpful for treating acne and eczema.

Added to fruit juices or sipped neat, aloe juice soothes and helps the digestive system recover from gastro-intestinal upsets. As a flower essence, aloe vera restores inner balance, helping to replenish the life energies and lift states of exhaustion. It is also known to mend holes in the aura.

Pineapple

LATIN NAME: *Ananas comosus*
FAMILY: *Bromeliaceae*

"My sweet juice nourishes the soul and helps man to absorb goodness from life."

This extraordinary plant bearing delicious golden fruits was once a symbol of welcome and hospitality. The spirit of pineapple is generous and nourishing, helping to enhance life in every way.

SPIRIT AND SYMBOLISM

With sweet fruits that grow from hundreds of tiny blossoms, the pineapple plant is laden with goodness and nourishment.

Growing wild along the sandy shores of South America and the West Indies, pineapple has long been valued as a medicinal plant. Native peoples make its fermented juice into an alcoholic drink for reducing

LEFT *The succulent juices of the pineapple have aided health for centuries.*

ORIGIN
Native to South America, the pineapple is cultivated throughout the tropics. It is prized both for its fruit and the fiber of the leaves.

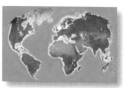

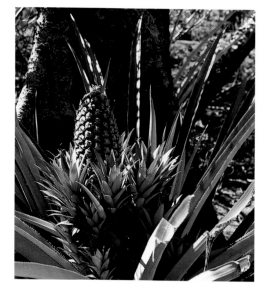

LEFT *The diverse properties of the pineapple plant are recognized throughout the world.*

fevers and cooling the body in hot weather. The juice is used externally to cure skin ailments and dissolve painful corns. The islanders of Guadaloupe applied pineapple flesh to wounds sustained in battle to promote rapid healing; they also made it into hair-removing preparations.

PLANT SPIRIT MEDICINES

Pineapple is a rich source of bromelain, a protein-digesting enzyme and anti-inflammatory agent. Compresses soaked in pineapple juice clean wounds and can help to treat sprains, strains, skin infections, and burns. In beauty treatments, it is a gentle exfoliator that clarifies, brightens, and softens the skin, but it is contraindicated for eczema. To enhance health, eat four slices of fresh pineapple or drink a glass of fresh pineapple juice every day. In Chinese medicine, pineapple is for fluid retention, indigestion, bloating, sickness, and diarrhea.

As a flower essence, pineapple promotes confidence, commitment, and a strong sense of identity. It brings self-assurance to those who constantly try to compare themselves to others, or are unhappy in their jobs and find themselves unable to follow a career path.

Angelica

LATIN NAME: *Angelica spp.*

FAMILY: *Umbelliferae*

"My gentle, yet strong energy helps a woman to go within and creates balance when in the world of spirits."

Angelic in name and nature, this plant embodies qualities of feminine strength and purity. Carrying clusters of pure white flowers, her spirit sits in balance between heaven and earth.

SPIRIT AND SYMBOLISM

An old legend claims the benefits of angelica were revealed to a monk by an angel. Though her spirit is strong and compassionate, angelica is a shy plant and she may be difficult to locate.

Angelica is a sacred medicine to Native Americans and shamans carried a stem of angelica to stay balanced when travelling in the spirit worlds. Known as arctic root in Scandinavia, folk belief holds that anyone finding angelica will be blessed with lifelong luck and health. Chinese emperors revered angelica as a treasured elixir of youth. In

ORIGIN
Angelica grows in damp sites in temperate regions ranging from Europe to the Himalayas and Siberia.

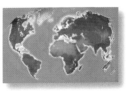

medieval times, angelica was seen as having supernatural powers against contagious diseases and Paracelsus burned the roots and seeds to purify the air during a sixteenth century epidemic in Milan. Today it is taken on a daily basis by women worldwide as a soothing tonic.

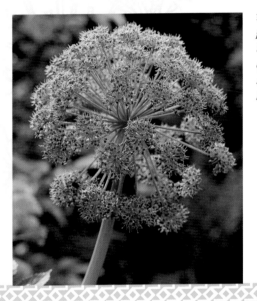

LEFT *Angelica produces striking ball-shaped clusters of flowers set on stems producing healing resources.*

PLANT SPIRIT MEDICINES

As an infusion of the whole plant, angelica normalizes the female reproductive system, stimulating delayed menstruation, soothing cramps, and easing symptoms of PMT and the menopause.

Steeped in brandy and drunk before or after meals, angelica root normalizes digestion, restores appetite, and lifts exhaustion. Chewing slices of dried root twice a day for six months builds resistance to viral infections.

Essential oil of angelica is a superb healer of scars, wounds, and bruises. As a flower

LEFT *Oils and infusions from angelica treat physical and emotional ailments.*

essence, angelica offers spiritual protection and guidance, and strengthens trust and resilience in difficult times or crises. A helpful remedy for emergencies when we feel our lives are threatened and for major life changes.

Wormwood

LATIN NAME: *Artemisia absinthium*
FAMILY: *Compositae*

"I am a psychic energizer and can stimulate lucid dreaming. I cleanse and knit together the subtle anatomy."

Known to Native Americans as desert sage or sage brush, wormwood is traditionally used in sacred ceremonies for its cleansing and purifying powers.

SPIRIT AND SYMBOLISM

Dedicated to Artemis, the ancient Greek goddess of fertility, this plant is also sacred to Native Americans. Living high in mountain valleys where the air is fresh and clean, the spirit of wormwood is crystal clear and serves to cleanse and knit together the subtle anatomy.

Native American elders have long revered wormwood's capacity to clear away negative thoughts and feelings to create a sacred space. It plays a part in almost every spiritual ceremony, especially the sundance, a form of initiation in which Blackfoot dancers tie this plant around their wrists and ankles. Wormwood is burned as an incense in the seven sacred rituals of the Sioux, including the purifying sweat lodge that symbolizes a dying of the old ways in order to be reborn afresh.

RIGHT *Wormwood has remained a valuable medicine, as used by the Blackfoot Native Indians.*

ORIGIN
Wormwood originates from the mainland and the islands of Greece, it also appears in the Americas.

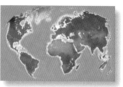

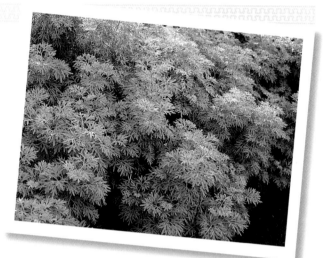

ABOVE *Wormwood is a prolific grower; it can easily run wild.*

PLANT SPIRIT MEDICINES

As a smudging agent wormwood is cut and gathered into a bundle, then dried before being burned to yield its cleansing and purifying smoke. In the sweat lodge the dried or moistened leaves are placed on hot stones and their vapor is inhaled and wafted over the body. As an infusion, wormwood tea is bitter and promotes sweating in feverishness, but due to the presence of thujone, a substance that affects the brain, it should only ever be taken in very small quantities.

Wormwood flower essence balances those susceptible to over–emotional and irrational behaviour. It gives insight into dreams to bring a deeper understanding of life.

Belladonna *or* Deadly Nightshade

LATIN NAME: *Atropa belladonna*

FAMILY: *Solanaceae*

"My magical essence protects you while you enter other realms."

A magical plant with two different dimensions – one medicinal, the other quite deadly – belladonna must be treated with caution and respect. She can open the doorway to other worlds, but warns of hidden dangers.

ORIGIN

Belladonna is native to Europe.

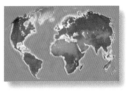

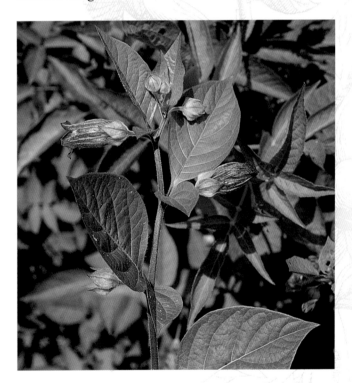

ABOVE *Handle with care – belladonna has much to offer if treated with respect.*

PLANT SPIRIT MEDICINES

Though belladonna may be deadly (the berries are a common cause of poisoning in children), this plant has great medicinal value. The active principles found in the leaves and root are a constituent of many pharmaceutical products and show promise for treating eye disease, peptic ulcers, and kidney stones. In homeopathic amounts, belladonna brings relief from violent headaches, throbbing pains, and infections accompanied by flushed skin, dilated pupils, and high fevers.

As a flower essence, she opens the third eye, our center of intuition and perception. She is

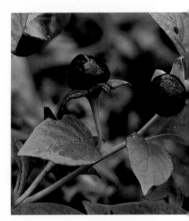

ABOVE *In spite of its name, deadly nightshade has a soothing effect on severe headaches.*

helpful during times of confusion and mental, emotional, and spiritual instability. A useful remedy for parents lacking insight who find themselves becoming intolerant, inappropriately strict, and constantly angry.

SPIRIT AND SYMBOLISM

Her flowers resemble lanterns, with the ability to open the eyes and bring spiritual illumination, but her dark berries are deadly poisonous. In Greek mythology, Atropos is one of the Fates, the one who cuts the thread of life. The name belladonna, meaning "beautiful lady," refers to the aristocratic ladies of Rome who dropped the juice of the berries into their eyes to make their pupils dilate, a sign of sexual arousal attractive to the opposite sex. In European folklore, belladonna was used magically as an ingredient in "flying" ointments. On May eve, the Germanic witches, or hexen, rubbed these psychedelic salves into their skin to initiate astral flights.

Neem

LATIN NAME: *Azadirachta indica*

FAMILY: *Meliaceae*

"I help you to tap into your ancient past to retrieve forgotten skills."

Native to India and Burma, the shady neem has been revered for centuries. Ancient Sanskrit writings sing the praises of this virtuous and versatile tree.

SPIRIT AND SYMBOLISM

Neem is a tall and splendid tree whose spreading branches provide a refuge from the blazing sun and biting insects. It bears a mass of honey-scented white flowers that give way to swollen fruits resembling olives. The spirit of neem is wise and knowing, helping us to learn from life's lessons. It was once worshipped in India and during special ceremonies neem was married to the sacred tree, *Ficus religiosa*. Thousand-year-old Sanskrit medical writings praise the virtues of its fruits, seeds, oils, and leaves, which all feature in the ancient Ayurvedic system of medicine. In Asia, neem is considered a

ORIGIN
The neem tree is native to India, Burma, and Africa.

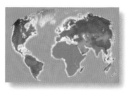

"cure all" for some childhood diseases, and for spotty diseases, like smallpox and chickenpox, leaves are rubbed directly onto the skin. Every morning millions of Indians break off a twig of neem, chew the end into a brush, and use it to scrub their teeth and gums.

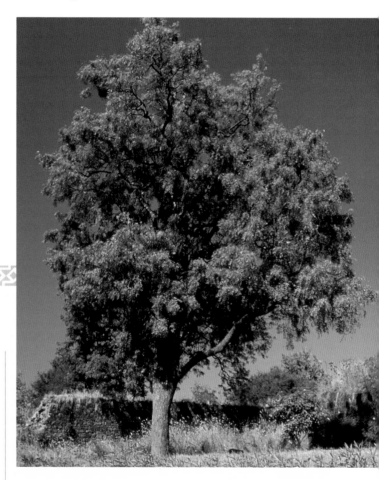

ABOVE *Standing proudly against a vivid blue sky, neem contains a host of cures.*

PLANT SPIRIT MEDICINES

The seeds and leaves of neem possess antiseptic, antiviral, and antifungal properties. As a poultice, the leaves help to treat boils, septic sores, and burns. An infusion of neem leaves and seeds is a strong insect repellent and prevents mosquito bites. It also kills the bacteria responsible for food poisoning and typhoid.

As an oil, neem can be rubbed into the skin to treat ringworm. Neem flower essence enables those who rationalize and think too much to become more intuitive, understanding, and less judgmental. It helps to enhance memory and may be used in past life recall.

Frankincense *or* Olibanum

LATIN NAME: *Boswellia carteri*
FAMILY: *Burseraceae*

"My sacred smoke purifies and frees the spirit."

At one time this richly perfumed resin was as valuable as gold, for the spirit of frankincense evokes the divine. Its sumptuous aroma warms the heart, clears the mind, and enables the spirit to soar.

SPIRIT AND SYMBOLISM

Frankincense is a golden gum that comes from the bark of *Boswellia*, a small tree bearing white or pale pink flowers. The name derives from *frank*, an Old French word meaning pure or free and the Latin *incensum*, to smoke.

ORIGIN
Frankincense comes from Malaysia, the Middle East, and North Africa.

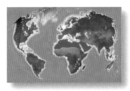

Frankincense focuses spiritual consciousness and evokes the potential for transcendent awareness. Native to the Middle East and North Africa, frankincense was used for religious purposes since earliest times. The ancient Egyptians worshipped the sun god Ra with frankincense, as did the Greeks their god Apollo. Herodotus recounts how 57,320 pounds/26,000kg of frankincense was burned on the golden altars of Babylon as an offering to Bael, another solar deity. Frankincense was Balthazar's offering to the infant Jesus and is a key ingredient of Jewish Sabbath-day incense.

LEFT *The gum from the bark of the Boswellia tree has been highly valued for thousands of years.*

PLANT SPIRIT MEDICINES

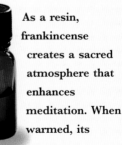

As a resin, frankincense creates a sacred atmosphere that enhances meditation. When warmed, its

ABOVE *Spiritual frankincense soothes and heals both the mind and the body.*

aroma purifies and uplifts the mind, body, and spirit.

Essential oil of frankincense has relaxing qualities that soothe nervous tension and alleviate exhaustion. When used in steam inhalations, frankincense eases the

congestion of sinusitis, laryngitis, and bronchitis.

In India, frankincense is an ancient remedy for rheumatic conditions, and an extract from *B. serrata* has excellent properties that reduce pain. It may be taken internally or applied as

a warm, soothing balm. As a beauty treatment, frankincense has been used by many historical beauties; it was known to the Egyptian queen Cleopatra and creams containing the essence have remarkable rejuvenating and rebalancing qualities.

Copal

LATIN NAME: *Bursera microphylla*

FAMILY: *Burseraceae*

"I create a smoking mirror that reveals all things."

Copal is a golden, black, or white resin whose sacred smoke carries messages to the spirit world. Its spirit inspires divine insights and allows us to see life more clearly.

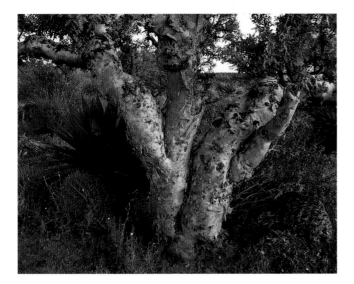

ABOVE *Nicknamed the "Elephant" tree, the bursera produces the magical resin used in Mayan ritual.*

SPIRIT AND SYMBOLISM

The sturdy *Bursera* tree grows wild on rocky outcrops in desert regions of southern Mexico. A milky liquid, which pours from the bark when cut, changes color as it hardens. To Mayan Indians, copal incense is very sacred, especially the resin that comes from trees struck by lightning or "Thunderbeings." They believe that this resin has a beautiful spirit.

In the Popul Vuh, a sacred book predating the Spanish conquest, copal is described as a "seeing instrument." Copal smoke reveals invisible energies that appear like rays of sunlight filtering through an early morning mist. In Hispanic communities today, copal incense is burnt on Dia de Los Muertos, the Day of the Dead, to sustain the departed on their journey into the spirit realm.

ORIGIN

The copal is originally from South America.

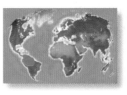

PLANT SPIRIT MEDICINES

Copal incense still burns at household altars and wayside shrines of Momostenango, Chichicastenango, and the holy mountain of Patohil to give nourishment to the gods. The smoke is used by the "day-keeper diviner," who casts lots of copal seeds and crystals along the traditional 260-day calendar. The amber-like aroma and chanting send him into a trance in which he receives images from the future. Healers use the copal smoke as a diagnostic tool to help them see the deeper dimensions of a client's energy field. They gaze through the smoke to detect illness and energy blocks.

Copal incense could be used in your sacred ceremony of thankfulness. Inhaling its mystical aroma works wonders for clearing and clarifying the mind.

BELOW *The Easter celebrations in Antigua include the swinging of copal incense.*

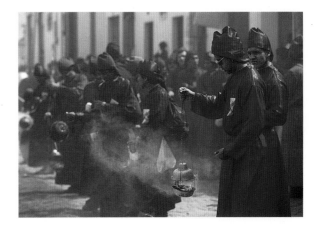

Marigold

LATIN NAME: *Calendula officinalis*
FAMILY: *Compositae*

"I bring the radiance and warmth of the sun into life, spiritually dissolving rigidity and materialism."

Sometimes known as "summer's bride," marigold embodies the warming and healing qualities of the sun's golden rays. The spirit of marigold inspires compassion, mellowness, and receptivity.

SPIRIT AND SYMBOLISM

A plant that enjoys basking in the sun, marigold's flowers are drenched in shades of the sunset. In Greek legend, Caltha fell in love with the sun god and when she was melted by his rays, a solitary marigold grew in her place. In English folklore, it is the flower of love and life-sustaining virtue. Following the sun across the sky, it symbolizes constancy and endurance in love. Marigold was woven into wedding garlands and love charms for luck, while its petals were placed in the mattress or under the bed to make dreams come true and added to bath water to attract respect and admiration.

Cut when the sun is at its highest, marigolds are said to act as a heart tonic and fortifier, a quality noted by the acclaimed herbalist, Culpeper. Arabs fortify their horses' feed with marigold to enhance endurance and make them swift of foot.

LEFT *An illustration from* Culpeper's Complete Herbal *c. 1820. All parts of the marigold can be used in healing remedies, and the young leaves even in salads.*

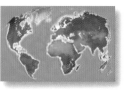

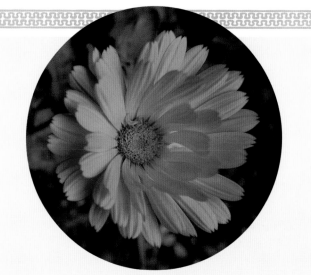

ABOVE *Not only beautiful, the marigold is a valuable medicinal plant.*

PLANT SPIRIT MEDICINES

An infusion of dried flowers calms itchy eyes and makes a wonderful toner for the skin. Sipping marigold tea can help pre-menstrual tension. As a golden oil added to creams and ointments, marigold heals bruising, sprains, wounds, and scar tissue.

Marigold essential oil, distilled from the flower tops, soothes sensitive skin and is good for burns. And as a homeopathic remedy, *Calendula* promotes the healing of wounds.

As a flower essence, marigold particularly enhances sensitivity and compassion, especially in communication with others. It encourages flexibility and clears away the materialistic view of life, permitting an opening to new and unexplored psychic and spiritual dimensions.

Tea

LATIN NAME: *Camellia sinensis*
FAMILY: *Theaceae*

"I bring mental alertness, brighten the mind, and stimulate easy communication."

The fresh green leaves of the tea plant provide one of the world's most delightful and ancient beverages. Grown on sunny mountain slopes throughout the tropics, this plant gives an impression of clarity and vitality.

SPIRIT AND SYMBOLISM

A lush bush with snowy white flowers, *Camellia sinensis* originates from the source of the Irawaddy River. The spirit of tea has a sparkling eloquence that conveys lightness and brightness. Tea has been sipped with reverence in China for some 2,000 years and many a tale is spun about its origins. One of the most popular tells how Bodhidharma, an Indian Prince and Brahmin, came to China to spread the word of Buddha. As an expression of piety he vowed not to sleep until his mission was accomplished, but after years of wakeful

ORIGIN
The tea bush is native to south east China and the region of the Irawaddy River.

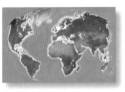

teaching, praying, and meditating, he succumbed. On waking he cut off his eyelids in an act of self-punishment and threw them to the ground, but Buddha made them sprout into the first tea shrub, a gift of eternal wakefulness.

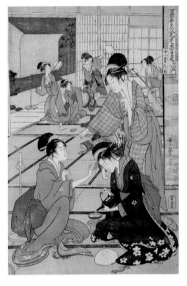

In Japan the tea ceremony is still performed with religious ritual to serve as a reminder of the once sacred use of this revitalizing brew.

LEFT *The ultimate Japanese tea ceremony, as depicted in a color woodblock print by Kitagawa Utamoro c. 1797.*

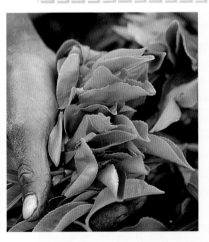

ABOVE *Picking the best of the tea crop at Labookellie estate in Sri Lanka.*

PLANT SPIRIT MEDICINES

An infusion of fermented black tea leaves wakes up the spirit, promotes digestion, and encourages mental focus and clarity. In Chinese medicine, tea is used for treating headaches, blurred vision, sleepiness, and excessive thirst.

Unfermented green tea, drunk in China and Japan, has remarkable anti-oxidant powers that offer protection from pollutants, speedy recovery from infections, and also lower blood pressure.

As a flower essence, tea stimulates

ABOVE *The necessary equipment to infuse the perfect cup of tea.*

creativity and helps overcome mental stagnation and lethargy.

Cedar

LATIN NAME: *Cedrus libani ssp. atlantica*
FAMILY: *Pinaceae*

"I bring a gift of abundant power coupled with spiritual strength."

This majestic tree has a powerful and protective spirit. Symbolizing abundance and spiritual strength, the cedar can help us to stand firm in the face of sudden danger and overwhelming emotions.

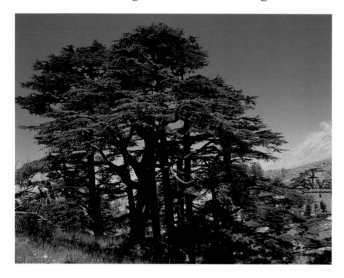

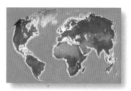

ORIGIN
Aromatic cedar is native to Morocco, Syria, and south east Turkey.

SPIRIT AND SYMBOLISM

One of the oldest known trees, cedar is a magnificent conifer whose spreading branches proffer shelter. Its reddish bark exudes a warm, reassuring aroma. Much mentioned in the Old Testament, it represented spiritual dignity and strength. King Solomon built his temples from the wood of cedar groves still found on the slopes of Mount Lebanon. Ancient Accadians living in Mesopotamia believed Ea, the name of their chief god, was inscribed upon their sacred cedar and in Babylon the tree was closely associated with the divine mother goddess, Ishtar.

Nordic peoples used cedar to invoke the spirit of Wotan, the one-eyed god of storm, magic, and harvest who inspires in us the fortitude to weather turbulent times and turn them to our advantage. In Arthurian legend, cedar consecrates the magic sword, a symbol of protection and courage.

LEFT *The mighty cedars of Lebanon dominate the landscape.*

PLANT SPIRIT MEDICINES

LEFT *Oil from the cedar promotes healthy hair.*

Experience the strong, protective energy of cedar by sitting in a bough of the tree. Inhale the warm aroma of the wood. The essential oil of cedar wood also fortifies and strengthens, making an excellent energy tonic and aid to poor concentration. The ancient Egyptians used it as incense to evoke the divine, as well as for its cosmetic qualities and fine perfume. It has a highly therapeutic action on the scalp for treating hair loss and dandruff, especially when due to illness and stress.

As a flower essence, cedar aids assimilation of strengthening nutrients and promotes elimination of toxins through the colon.

Camomile

LATIN NAME: *Chamaemelum nobile (common or Roman camomile),*
Matricaria recutita (wild or German camomile)

FAMILY: *Compositae*

"I bring you the gift of a calm, sunny disposition."

There is perhaps no flower that soothes the psyche like camomile. Modest daisy-like flowers belie camomile's strong spirit. For above all, this little plant represents an ability to stay cool and collected in the face of adversity.

SPIRIT AND SYMBOLISM

With its distinctive aroma of newly mown hay, camomile reminds us of relaxing summer days. To ancient Egyptians, camomile represented the omnipotence of the sun god Ra. Camomile was used to invoke this solar deity and for medicinal purposes. To the Druids it brought the power of the sun to their potions and spells. Shakespeare said of camomile "the more it is trodden, the faster it grows," recognizing its ability to help us cope with adversity.

ORIGIN
Camomile grows profusely across Europe and is native to North Africa.

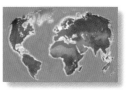

PLANT SPIRIT MEDICINES

As a herbal tincture or tisane, camomile soothes nervous indigestion, stomach upset, and headaches. Sip a cup of camomile tea at bedtime to promote a good night's sleep and prevent nightmares. Used as a beauty treatment, a camomile rinse brings golden lights to fair hair. The essential oil of camomile owes its pale bluish tinge to an anti-inflammatory chemical called azulene that promotes rapid healing of skin problems and wounds. One of the gentlest essential oils, it is safe to use for babies and children with eczema and irritable skin conditions.

As a homeopathic remedy, camomile treats childhood conditions, such as teething and colic, when little ones are tearful and hard to console.

As a flower essence, camomile eases emotional stress in the nervous system and solar plexus. It calms and releases anxiety and fear in those who are easily upset and who harbor emotional tension in the stomach.

BELOW *Camomile is used in the treatment of stomach disorders.*

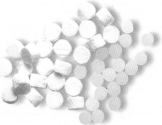

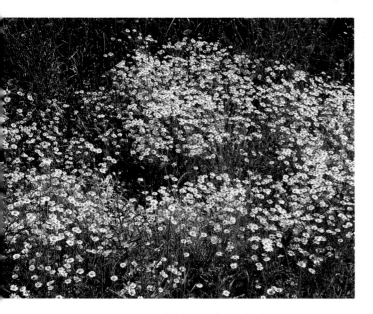

ABOVE *Wild camomile growing in profusion. Flower heads should be harvested when the white petals turn down.*

Chrysanthemum

LATIN NAME: *Chrysanthemum spp.*

FAMILY: *Compositae*

"My elixir of life promotes longevity."

In their many shades of autumnal gold, chrysanthemums bring color into lives as well as ornamental gardens. The spirit of this flower brings warmth and comfort, especially to those in the autumn of life.

ORIGIN
China is home to the chrysanthemum.

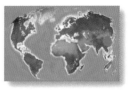

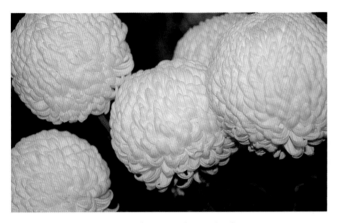

ABOVE *The chrysanthemum has been bred into many wonderful varieties, such as this incurved one.*

SPIRIT AND SYMBOLISM

Chrysanthemums originally come from China, where these golden flowers are known as Queen of the Fall. Cultivated in Chinese gardens for more than 2,500 years, they were assigned with scholarly qualities after the fourth century poet T'ao Yuan-Ming retired from government office to spend time with his beloved chrysanthemums.

According to Chinese legend, an Emperor of China heard chrysanthemums promised an elixir of life if picked by the pure of heart, so he dispatched three hundred virginal youths to search for these flowers. As one might expect, the virgins lost their purity along the way and the Emperor never acquired immortality.

In the Mediterranean, *Chrysanthemum coronarium* was used to make garlands worn as protection against demonic spirits. In France they are still associated with Halloween.

PLANT SPIRIT MEDICINES

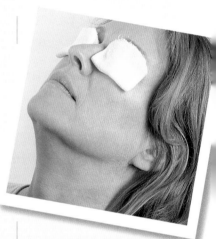

An infusion of chrysanthemum flowers is used in Chinese medicine in a manner similar to camomile or marigold. It is a cooling herb that helps to tone the liver, lower blood pressure, soothe inflammation, and relieve eye problems. Pieces of muslin soaked in this solution make good eye pads for sore, irritated eyes.

ABOVE *The soothing effect of an infusion of chrysanthemum brings relief to tired eyes.*

As a flower essence, chrysanthemum calms the emotions and helps to dispel irritation and lift depression. It is a remedy that enables a person to open up emotionally in the right circumstances, such as when grieving.

LEFT *The beauty of the versatile chrysanthemum is portrayed in this exquisite watercolor.*

Cinnamon

LATIN NAMES: *Cinnamomum verum*
FAMILY: *Lauracea*

"I help to express beauty that comes from the heart."

Cinnamon is a treasured spice, well loved for its warm and enriching qualities. The spirit of cinnamon sets the heart aglow, encouraging clearer expression of our innermost feelings.

SPIRIT AND SYMBOLISM

Though the yellow flowers, fruits, leaves, and roots of this evergreen tree all boast cinnamon's rich aroma, the spice comes from its sepia-colored bark. An ancient spice, cinnamon was mentioned almost 5,000 years ago in the works of the Emperor Shen Nung, the founder of Chinese herbal medicine. It is still one of most popular remedies in China.

ORIGIN
Cinnamon is a native of South East Asia and Sri Lanka.

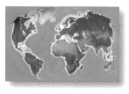

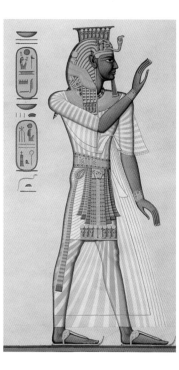

The ancient Egyptians were especially fond of cinnamon. Ramses III gave cinnamon to his high priests to use as gifts for Amun, their chief deity, and a fresco on the tomb of Queen Nefertari in Thebes depicts the burning of cinnamon incense. It was used to ward off infections and for embalming. Along with myrrh, olive oil, and bulrushes, Moses took valuable cinnamon with him when he fled Egypt for the promised land.

LEFT *Portrait of Ramses III.*

PLANT SPIRIT MEDICINES

As a spice, cinnamon has warming and stimulating qualities. In Chinese medicine it is used to treat cold, damp conditions with a predominance of yin energy. Adding cinnamon powder to milky drinks helps to relieve winter colds, sore throats, and coughs. Chewing a stick of cinnamon helps to freshen the breath and aids digestion after meals. The smell of cinnamon from candles containing its oil gives a room a warm and welcoming atmosphere.

Cinnamon essential oil, extracted from the leaves and bark, is strongly antiseptic but should be used only by a practitioner. As a flower essence, it balances the heart

ABOVE *Cinnamon sticks can be chewed to promote fresh breath and as an aid to digestion.*

chakra and enables one to articulate feelings that come from the heart. It can help introverts who have difficulty expressing their feelings.

Sturt's Desert Pea

LATIN NAME: *Clianthus formosus*
FAMILY: *Leguminosae*

"My tremendous strength gives you the power to release all pain, initiate profound change, and start afresh."

With delicate flowers of the brightest blood-red color, Sturt's desert pea grows in the heart of Australia. Held with great reverence by the native Aborigines, it symbolizes the eternal ability to bloom in the face of adversity.

SPIRIT AND SYMBOLISM

The most spectacular of native plants, Sturt's desert pea is the floral emblem of South Australia. Its spirit has a powerful and commanding presence, with the ability to trigger the cathartic release of deep-seated hurt. Old Aboriginal tribes refer to Sturt's desert pea as the flower of blood, symbolizing the ancestral blood spilt in their struggle for survival.

RIGHT *The intensity of the bright red flowers of Sturt's desert pea illuminates the arid landscape.*

ORIGIN
A native of Australia, Sturt's desert pea is sacred to the Aborigine tribes.

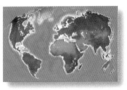

Their legends tells the story of Wimbaco, a man who eloped with a woman called Purleemil, betrothed to Tirtha. The couple were welcomed by a tribe living by a lake and Purleemil gave birth to a son. One tragic night, the embittered Tirtha and his men massacred the whole tribe. The lake then turned to salt. A mass of brilliant red flowers grew where the bodies had lain and a heavenly voice said: "Their blood shall live forever, for it will bloom along the bare plains of the salt lakes, which are the dried tears of the song spirits."

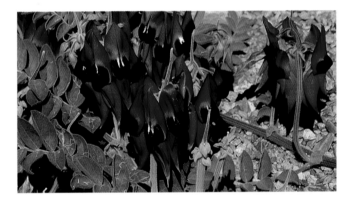

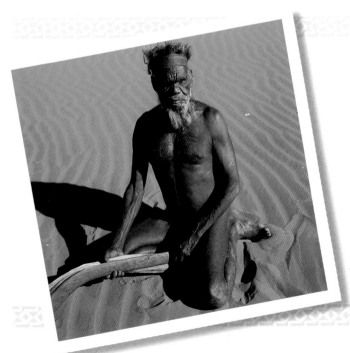

PLANT SPIRIT MEDICINES

To sense the spirit of this flower, it is best to sit among them, as the aborigines do, and allow their strength and courage to flow through you.

LEFT *Sturt's desert pea plays an integral part in the lives of the Aboriginal people.*

As a flower essence, Sturt's desert pea eases pain, deep hurt, and sadness. It encourages the cathartic release of sad memories and feelings and provides the motivation and energy to bring about positive change.

Coconut

LATIN NAME: *Cocos nucifera*
FAMILY NAME: *Palmae*

"My sweet milk uplifts, nourishes, and helps one to endure life."

There is no tree that captures the essence of tropical paradise quite like the swaying coconut palm. A symbol of bounty, the coconut holds the promise of a sweeter life.

SPIRIT AND SYMBOLISM

In the words of an old South Sea proverb, "He who plants a coconut tree, plants food and drink, vessels and clothing, a habitation for himself and a heritage for his children." The spirit of coconut reminds us that nature provides for all our spiritual needs.

Like umbrellas, coconut palms line most tropical shores since the fruits are carried with the tides. Coconuts may have originated in the Melanesian area of the Pacific. In creation stories of these islands, To-Karvuvu gathers coconuts and dashes them to pieces. Two women then emerge to become the wives of himself and To-Kabinana, the first humans to walk upon the earth.

Coconuts are much revered by Hawaiians, who know them as niu. Their legends tell of a magical coconut palm that is discovered by a Hawaiian queen and which carries her to heaven to be reunited with her grandfather.

ORIGIN
The coconut is abundant in the southern Pacific.

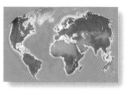

PLANT SPIRIT MEDICINES

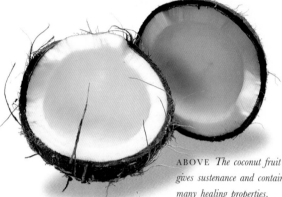

ABOVE *The coconut fruit gives sustenance and contains many healing properties.*

The coconut fruit has nourishing and healing qualities. Rich in vitamin C, amino acids, and minerals, its clear juice or "milk" is used to treat sore throats, stomach upsets, sunstroke, edema, and sickness. Its white meat, rich in the mineral iodine, keeps the thyroid gland healthy and is renowned for destroying intestinal worms.

As a flower essence, coconut (niu) is uplifting and inspires the endurance to meet any kind of challenge. It stimulates a mother's instinct to breastfeed, helps balance male and female energies, and brings clarity in issues of sexuality.

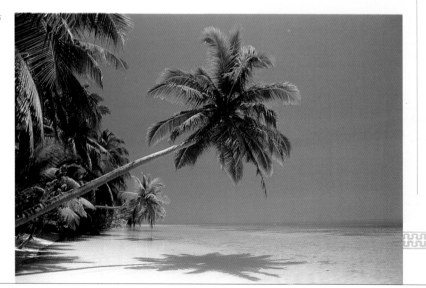

RIGHT *Everybody's dream of paradise. The coconut tree symbolises pure sand, clear seas, and uninterrupted sunshine, but its fruit provides much more.*

Coffee

LATIN NAME: *Coffea arabica*

FAMILY: *Rubiaceae*

"I offer a gift of acute alertness, accompanied by a sense of calm and stability."

Native originally to Ethiopia, coffee is now known and beloved throughout the world. Nestling inside the crimson coffee berries are small green beans with amazing powers to spark creative inspiration, sharpen the mind, and enhance physical stamina.

SPIRIT AND SYMBOLISM

Like its white star-shaped flowers and glossy green leaves, the spirit of coffee is clear and bright. Coffee comes from the ancient Abyssinian province of Caffa, where its uplifting and energizing qualities have been known to the indigenous people since time immemorial.

In Ethiopian legend, a goatherd called Kaldi noticed how lively his flock became after nibbling berries from a certain shrub. He tried a few himself and felt so wonderfully awake that he told the chief mullah, who claimed these berries were just what he needed to keep the faithful awake. And so coffee became a sacred beverage. In ancient times, roasted and ground coffee beans were mixed with grease to make balls of food for Abyssinian warriors to keep them alert and energized during a battle.

ORIGIN

The coffee plant hails from north-east Africa.

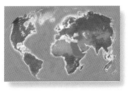

PLANT SPIRIT MEDICINES

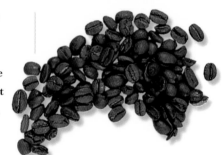

Simply inhaling the aroma of freshly ground coffee can warm and uplift the spirits. As a drink it awakens, energizes, and allows us to reach beyond our normal limits of capability. In Chines medicine, coffee has warm, sweet, and bitter qualities helpful in treating bronchitis, fluid retention, and sluggish circulation.

As a homeopathic remedy, *Coffea cruda* can dampen over-excitement and sensitivity, but like the drink, it can negate the effects of other homeopathic remedies. As a flower essence, coffee has a cleansing and stabilizing effect on the parasympathetic nervous system, reducing the physical and nervous instability which leads to a craving for coffee. Take a few drops for decisiveness and inspiration.

LEFT *The coffee plant growing in Paraná State in Brazil, a major coffee-producing area of the world.*

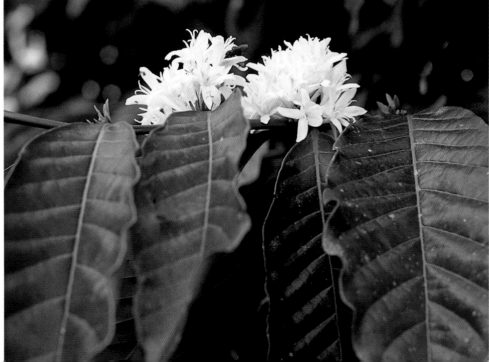

Myrrh

LATIN NAME: *Commiphora myrrha*
FAMILY: *Burseraceae*

*"I will accompany you on your soul's journey.
I bridge the divide between heaven and earth."*

Like frankincense, myrrh has always been seen as a sacred substance. In ancient times it was worth its weight in gold. The spirit of myrrh spins ethereal threads that link the physical and spiritual realms.

SPIRIT AND SYMBOLISM

Myrrh comes from a thorny shrub bearing small white flowers that grows in the Middle East, North Africa, and Northern India. Prized for its opulent and enduring perfume, myrrh was seen as a magical substance that was capable of connecting heaven and earth.

To the ancient Egyptians, the golden drops of myrrh that solidify to chestnut-

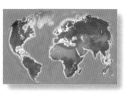

ORIGIN
Myrrh is a native of Arabia, the Middle East, North Africa, and India.

colored resin were the tears of Horus, their falcon-headed sun god. Known as punt or phun, myrrh was included in their sacred perfume Kyphi, burned at sunset as a thanksgiving to the sun god Ra. Used during funerals and in embalming, myrrh was thought to accompany the soul on its journey to the spirit world. When Moses left Egypt he took myrrh with him. The Hebrews drank wine flavored with myrrh to prepare them for worship. One of the three gifts to infant Jesus, myrrh also featured at His death, when Nicodemus anointed His body with a mixture of myrrh and aloes.

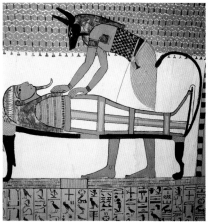

LEFT *Anubis, the jackal-headed god of the dead and god of embalmers – a wall painting from the tomb of Tutankhamun c. 1361–52 B.C.E.*

PLANT SPIRIT MEDICINES

Burned as incense, myrrh strengthens the link between our crown and base chakras. Its perfume evokes tranquility, calms the nervous system, and eases sorrow and grief by helping to heal the wounds caused by the feelings of loss and rejection.

As an essential oil, myrrh has wonderful skin-healing properties. It is added to ointments and salves to clear scars, infections, and problems such as acne and dermatitis. Combined with mint essential oil, myrrh makes an effective

antiseptic mouthwash for gum problems, mouth ulcers, an sore throats, wh in steam inhal myrrh helps t relieve sinus

RIGHT *A di myrrh promotes heat... and induces calm.*

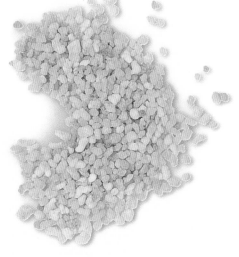

Ti

LATIN NAME: *Cordyline terminalis*
FAMILY: *Liliaceae*

ORIGIN
The most important plant in Hawaii, the ti bush originates from the Polynesian Islands.

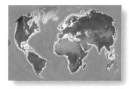

"By surrounding you with my spiritual light, my powerful energy clears and offers protection from psychic interference."

One of the most revered plants in Hawaii, ti bushes are traditionally planted around houses and temples for spiritual protection. Bearing clusters of tiny white flowers tinged with lilac, this plant provides shelter and refuge from all forms of negative energy.

SPIRIT AND SYMBOLISM

Polynesians so valued their native ti that these plants travelled with them when they set off to colonize the Hawaiian islands. Ti plants are believed to ward off evil spirits and today they still surround homes and temples to create a sanctuary of peace and harmony. The plant was dedicated to the God of agriculture, Lono, and legends tell how ti leaves were used in the Mahiki ritual conducted by a Kahuna-pule (priest) and Kahuna-lapa'au (doctor) to cast out evil spirits. Both Kahunas wore garlands of ti flowers and carried ti leaves as the sacred symbol of the Gods.

Ti plays a pivotal role in Hawaiian culture, with its leaves being used to serve and wrap food, thatch houses, and even make raincoats.

LEFT *Both the leaves and the flowers of the plant are used in a wide range of remedies.*

PLANT SPIRIT MEDICINES

In Hawaii, ti flowers and leaves are traditionally prepared as teas for alleviating asthma. Ti leaves are also moistened with cold water and applied as poultices to relieve headaches and fevers. Hot lava rocks wrapped in ti leaves make warm packs for soothing back pain.

As a flower essence, ti offers protection from invasive astral spirits and other forms of negative energy. This remedy is good for psychically stressed environments, such as the tension-charged work place, and for lifting a spell or curse put upon a place.

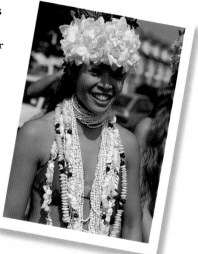

RIGHT *Known as the good luck plant, the ti bush yields flowers used in traditional Hawaiian costumes to dispel evil.*

Hawthorn *or* Maytree

LATIN NAME: *Crataegus laevigata*
FAMILY: *Rosaceae*

*"I am a 'path finder.' I will help you listen
to your heart and discover your path in life."*

The hawthorn has always been seen as a magical tree. With her snowy white flowers and bright red berries, hawthorn protects and nurtures the heart and in so doing sets the spirit free.

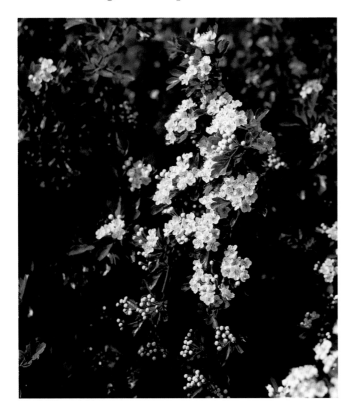

ORIGIN
*The trees of hawthorn can
be found all over Europe.*

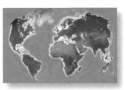

PLANT SPIRIT MEDICINES

The leaves, berries, and blossoms of hawthorn contain compounds believed to protect and strengthen the heart. As a tincture, hawthorn improves circulation in the blood vessels of the heart, reduces blood pressure, and enhances the use of life-sustaining oxygen.

As a flower essence, hawthorn protects the heart in times of extreme stress, pain, or grief. It stimulates the healing power of love and cleanses the heart of negativity to restore hope, trust, and forgiveness. Use this extract to free the spirit and follow your own path in life.

LEFT *In various forms the hawthorn is used as a medicine for the heart.*

LEFT *A welcome sight after a long winter, the hawthorn blossom signifies spring.*

SPIRIT AND SYMBOLISM

Like others in the rose family, hawthorn has a natural affinity with the heart. When dressed in her spring gown of white blossom, she signifies spiritual rebirth and the beauty it can bring. In folklore, hawthorn is much loved by fairies, who dance around this tree in joyful celebration at certain times of the year. Hawthorn may have been the original maypole, a symbol of fertility and the rebirth of life.

Hawthorn supposedly grew from a branch of the Holy Thorn that featured in the mystical tales of Joseph of Arimathea's travels. It is said that, after leaving the Holy Land, he came to Glastonbury, in England. There, he thrust his staff into the ground, where it took root, burst into leaf, and became the Holy Thorn, a tree which blossoms twice a year, once in spring and again at midnight on the 6th January, the original Christmas day.

Angel's Trumpet *and* Thorn Apple

LATIN NAME: *Datura inoxia and D. stramonium*
FAMILY: *Solanaceae*

"With my angel's trumpet I bring messages from angelic realms."

In shades of salmon, gold, and white, the angel's trumpet from Hawaii and its Peruvian cousin, the thorn apple, are perfectly shaped for heralding spirit messages. These beautiful flowers enhance our perception of the spirit world.

PLANT SPIRIT MEDICINES

The leaves and seeds of *Datura* contain hyoscyamine and hyoscine, powerful chemicals used medically as pre-anesthetic relaxants and as drugs for treating motion sickness. Herbal preparations are too dangerous to use at home as they are hallucinogenic in large doses.

As a homeopathic remedy, thorn-apple (**D. stramonium**) is indicated for anxiety, confusion, a sense of unreality, and fear of the dark, often following shock or childbirth. As a flower essence, angel's trumpet is completely safe and allows us to attune to the angelic realms for soul guidance, clarity of thought, and sharpness of mind.

BELOW *The Peruvian thorn apple has long had mystic powers and as a remedy, it calms and soothes.*

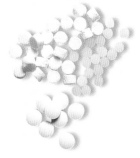

ORIGIN
The angel's trumpet plant originates from the Pacific Islands.

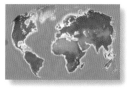

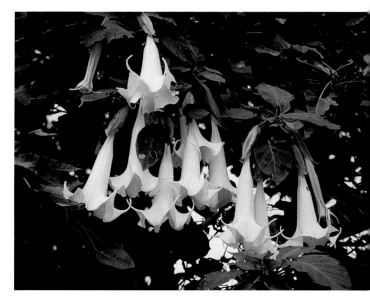

ABOVE *The angel's trumpet heralds a sharp mind and spiritual peace.*

SPIRIT AND SYMBOLISM

The spirit of *Datura* facilitates our ability to attune to the devas and nature spirits, a quality known to native Hawaiians and Peruvian Indians. It is said that thorn apple, or jimson-weed, is the descendant of a boy and girl who eavesdropped on the sacred council of spirits. When the children told their parents what they had seen and heard, the spirits were so angry that they changed them into *Datura* plants. By partaking of this plant, others can listen to the secrets of the spirits.

In Peru, a person praying for rain will chew on a piece of thorn apple root obtained from his shaman to call upon the spirits. In ancient times, Hawaiians smoked the leaves of the angel's trumpet for its hallucinogenic effects and in South American tribes the medicine men have used thorn apple as an anesthetic and narcotic medicine for generations. In the Far East, dried *Datura* leaves are traditionally smoked as cigarettes and burned as smoke candles to alleviate the symptoms of asthma.

Yam

LATIN NAME: *Dioscorea spp.*
FAMILY: *Discoreaceae*

ORIGIN
*The yam is native to
South America and Africa.*

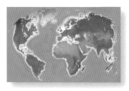

*"I am the food that bestows
timeless youth and vigor."*

**From this uninspiring brown
tuber grow clambering leafy
shoots reminiscent of the
fairy-tale beanstalk. The
spirit of yam embodies our
aspirations to live a long,
yet youthful, life.**

SPIRIT AND SYMBOLISM

Yams are valued throughout West
Africa, the Caribbean, and South
East Asia as a nourishing and health-
enhancing food. The native people
of Trobriand Island in New Guinea
stay amazingly youthful all their
lives, free from the degenerative
diseases associated with old age.

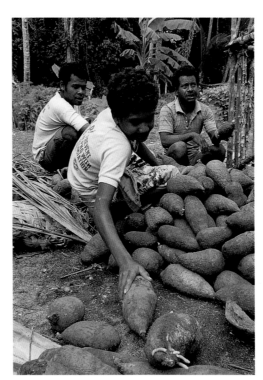

They attribute their radiant health to
eating yams.

In 25 B.C.E. the Mexican yam was
recorded in the Chinese *Pen Tsao
Ching* as a highly valued herb, and
medicine men in China, as well as
Central and South America, used
yams to treat female problems and for
birth control.

In West Africa, important ceremonies mark the beginning of the
yam season. The Fon priests make
offerings to the gods and ancestral
spirits to symbolize annual purification and renewal.

LEFT *Grading the crop – the yam
is an essential food, but it is also
valuable for its healing powers.*

PLANT SPIRIT MEDICINES

Yams can be eaten
boiled, fried, or
roasted. They are a
rich source of phyto-
hormones, which are
helpful for alleviating
menstrual and
menopausal symptoms,
such as hot flushes,
mood changes, and
sleep disruption, fluid
retention and weight

gain. Yams may also
help to treat breast
cysts and fibroids.
When yam essences
are added to creams,
the phyto-hormones
may be absorbed
through the skin.

In Chinese medicine,
yams are neutral and
sweet, a tonic for the
lungs, kidneys, and

spleen. Yam tea is
prescribed to
sustain well-being
and health from
maturity to graceful
old age. As a
homeopathic remedy,
wild yam is for
colicky pain with
cramping and
griping, especially
in babies.

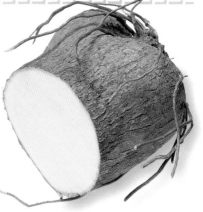

ABOVE *Eaten, used as
a healing cream, infused
as a tea – the yam is
highly versatile.*

Purple Cone Flower

ORIGIN
The North American purple cone flower originated in the Americas.

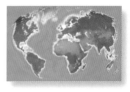

LATIN NAME: *Echinacea angustifolia*
FAMILY: *Compositae*

"My gift is to maintain the integrity of mind, body, and spirit."

With its daisy-like purple flowers, *Echinacea* is one of the Native Americans' most important medicines. Now widely valued for its immune-enhancing powers, the spirit of this flower draws all the systems together so they act in perfect harmony.

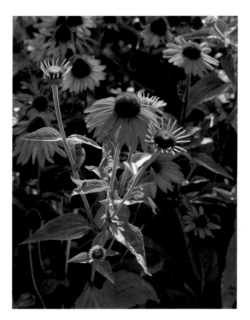

RIGHT *The purple cone flower in bloom. An infusion will soothe a bad throat.*

SPIRIT AND SYMBOLISM

Growing wild on the prairies and sandy banks of southern North America, the purple cone flower has been used as a medicine for generations by at least fourteen indigenous tribes. It is seen as a general purifier with the power to heal colds, coughs, inflammations, and cramps. Roots are often sucked all day to allay an imminent cold. *Echinacea* was introduced to Africa some 150 years ago and is often prescribed by African healers as an ointment or poultice for wounds to prevent them becoming septic and to promote healing.

PLANT SPIRIT MEDICINES

The whole plant strengthens and supports the immune system and should only be taken for up to ten days for a specific reason, for example at the first signs of a cold. An infusion or tincture of

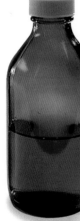

LEFT *Purple cone flower essence will calm a stressed body and mind.*

purple cone flower enhances resistance to viral attack and soothes a sore "strep" throat. It clears blemishes by cleansing the skin from within. Compresses soaked in this infusion or tincture are good for slow-healing wounds, mild burns, and abscesses. In healing salves or ointments, *Echinacea* encourages torn ligaments to heal by speeding tissue repair. When combined with St. John's wort it is particularly good for scarring.

As a flower essence, *Echinacea* aids recovery from shock and trauma which shatters the whole system. It brings complete reintegration of mind, body, and

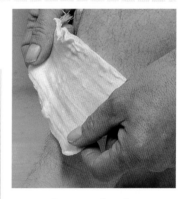

ABOVE *A compress of purple cone flower infusion for wounds and burns.*

spirit, so restoring a sense of dignity and identity and fortifying defences on all levels.

Cardamom

LATIN NAME: *Elattaria cardamomum*
FAMILY: *Zingiberaceae*

*"I am a reminder of true abundance
and contentment with life."*

**Cardamom evokes the colorfulness of its native
country. Prized for its peppery perfume and
medicinal properties, cardamom symbolizes
an appetite for the spice of life.**

SPIRIT AND SYMBOLISM

The tiny piquant cardamom seeds are packed into leathery
pods, the fruit of a plant that grows wild in the monsoon
forests of southern India and Sri Lanka.
Cardamom's yellowish
flowers with their violet lips
are said to resemble mouths
open in anticipation.
Cardamom is one of the
most ancient culinary
spices in the world. Known
in India as grains of
paradise, the seeds have
been valued for their
aromatic and medic-

ABOVE *Discard the pods
to release the minute seeds
used in a variety of cures.*

inal properties for centuries. The ancient
Sanskrit texts refer to cardamom or "ela"
as being hot and penetrating, qualities
that were harnessed by the Hindu
system of Ayurvedic medicine. Coated
in sugar, they are still used at Hindu
festivals and ceremonies. The Egyptians,
who adopted many medicines from
India, added cardamom to their
perfumes and used it in their religious
ceremonies. When introduced to
Greece, cardamom was warmly
embraced by Hippocrates, who
was delighted by its exquisite
aroma and therapeutic powers.

ORIGIN
*Cardamom originates from India
and Sri Lanka.*

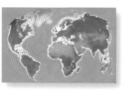

PLANT SPIRIT MEDICINES

In India, cardamom
seeds are traditionally
used to spice up every
aspect of life. As well
as adding warm and
piquant flavors to
cooking (cardamom is
an essential ingredient
of curry powder), the
seeds are prized for
their aphrodisiac
powers. They can be
made into a spicy
beverage by boiling
in a little water. When
chewed after
meals,

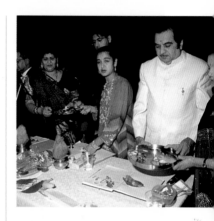

ABOVE *Cardamom is an
integral part of Indian cuisine.*

they aid digestion and
help to freshen the
breath.

As an essential oil,
cardamom has gentle
tonic properties that
help to fortify the body.
It is also a good
diuretic. Massaged into
the body, it can help
relieve fluid retention
that occurs around the
time of periods.

LEFT *An infusion of cardamom
produces a warming, spicy
drink, stimulating a sense of
well-being.*

Coca

LATIN NAME: *Erythroxylum coca*
FAMILY: *Erythroxylaceae*

"My gift is to bring a sense of sacredness to all your ceremonies and prayers."

One of the most ancient and esteemed of Peruvian medicines, coca is traditionally used in a sacred way to honor Mother Earth and re-establish one's place in the great web of life.

ORIGIN
The coca plant is a native of Peru and Bolivia.

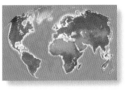

PLANT SPIRIT MEDICINES

Coca leaves contain the chemical cocaine which, when extracted and purified, has powerful narcotic and stimulating properties, making it an illegal substance. Scattered to the winds, coca leaves bring a sacredness to ceremonies and prayers. As a homeopathic remedy, coca helps combat the symptoms associated with altitude sickness. Coca flower essence reinvigorates, increases stamina, balances the appetite and metabolism, and brings a sense of joy.

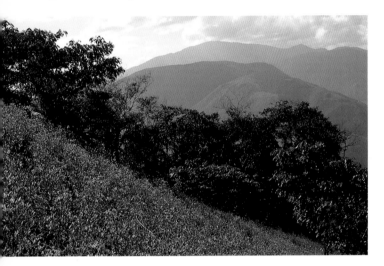

ABOVE *Coca growing in the mountains of South America, as it has for centuries.*

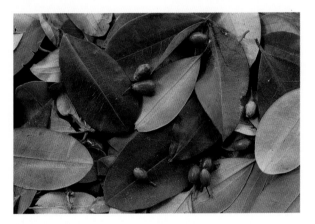

ABOVE *Coca leaves and berries.*

SPIRIT AND SYMBOLISM

The silvery green leaves of the coca plant mirror its spirit's lively and hedonistic nature. People of Peru have known and revered the energizing and mind-expanding qualities of coca for centuries. Bags for coca leaves and the iliptu, or lime, used for leaf chewing have been found in 4,500-year-old Peruvian graves.

The Incas considered coca sacred and the Despacho ceremony, still performed by their descendants, hints of its ancient use. In a traditional ritual for honoring "Pachamama" (sacred Mother Earth), the "kurak" draws a fistful of coca leaves from his pouch and utters a prayer to their spirit before letting them fall on his ceremonial tools. Participants share the coca leaves in a sacred act of spiritual and energetic bonding.

Confined to priestly and noble castes before the Spanish conquest, coca was used medicinally as an analgesic and early anesthetic. Natives of Peru and Bolivia still chew coca leaves to overcome the fatigue and dizziness of altitude sickness, although they rarely become addicted to them.

Fig

LATIN NAME: *Ficus carica*

FAMILY: *Moraceae*

"Under my sacred bough gain spiritual fluidity and light."

Sit beneath a fig tree and see the sun's rays filtering through its sculptured leaves to form ever-changing patterns on the ground. In contemplation, this tree brings divine inspiration. Deep purple fruits with blood-red flesh symbolize spiritual prosperity and fertility.

SPIRIT AND SYMBOLISM

Pips of these fruit-bearing trees have been found in early Neolithic sites dating back to 7,800 B.C.E. Fig trees were cultivated in Mesopotamia and Egypt almost 5,000 years ago and apparently grew in the Garden of Eden, since Adam and Eve covered their nakedness with its leaves. Its fruits symbolize

ORIGIN

The fig originates from the southern Mediterranean.

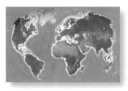

the feminine and fertile aspects of the earth goddess, while also hinting slightly of the erotic.

From the same family, *Ficus religiosa*, or the pipal, is one of the most sacred trees of India and was once worshipped as the home of the Hindu triad, Brahma, Vishnu, and Shiva. Charms of pipal wood were said to destroy enemies, secure the birth of male children, and bring healing. Close cousins are the banyan, or *F. indica*, a tree sacred to Vishnu, and the Bodhi, or Bo-Tree, at Buddh Gaya, reputedly the oldest and wisest tree in the world that for a while sheltered Gautama, the Buddha, as he received enlightenment.

LEFT Adam and Eve in the Garden of Eden, *oil on panel by Lucas Cranach the Elder (1472–1553).*

PLANT SPIRIT MEDICINES

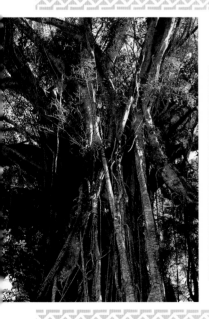

LEFT *The Curtain Fig, Tableland National Park, Queensland, Australia.*

The fruits are many times richer in minerals than most, making them ideal energy snacks. Soak fresh quartered figs in a syrup of honey overnight for a delicious dessert.

Their juice gently relieves constipation and soothes sore throats and coughs.

As a flower essence, the spirit of fig encourages flexibility in those who are strict, uncompromising, and have unrealistic expectations of themselves. It helps

RIGHT *Tasty and beneficial to eat, the fig produces extract promoting calm emotions.*

one to cope with the complexity of modern life in a calm, assured manner, dispelling hidden fears and resolving relationship conflicts.

Licorice

LATIN NAME: *Glycyrrhiza glabra*
FAMILY: *Leguminosae*

"I have the ability to soothe a restless spirit."

With its sweet comforting taste, licorice is one of the most ancient and widely used plant remedies. Its spirit helps to pacify and instill a sense of calmness at every level of one's being.

SPIRIT AND SYMBOLISM

Licorice is quite a common plant with pale lilac flowers and long running roots of yellow fibrous wood that yield the familiar, syrupy tasting licorice sticks. It grows throughout Europe, Russia, and the Middle East, with wild cousins in North America, China, and Mongolia.

Licorice was being used medicinally nearly 4,000 years ago, for it features in the Code of Hammarubi as part of the Mesopotamian pharmacy. It was favored by the great Arabian herbalists in medieval

ORIGIN
Licorice hails from the Mediterranean.

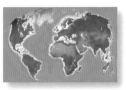

times and nomadic Bedouins still boil licorice root in water to make a strong decoction for relieving fevers. Licorice is esteemed in Chinese medicine and included in most prescriptions for common ills.

Folktales claim licorice brings fidelity and passion to sexual relations, so it was frequently added to lust spells and love potions. Licorice was also used for making magic wands.

LEFT *A plant of many parts* – Licorice, *a colored engraving by Werner in the 19th century.*

BELOW *The roots of the licorice plants make tasty chewing sticks.*

PLANT SPIRIT MEDICINES

Licorice's sweet taste comes from glycyrrhin, a substance fifty times sweeter than sugar with added medicinal properties. Its root may be chewed or a licorice juice obtained by boiling. Licorice soothes coughs, acts as

LEFT *The attractive licorice flowers produce a soothing extract.*

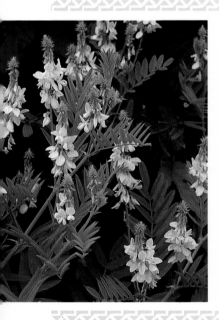

an expectorant, clearing congestion in the lungs, and helps to heal gastric ulcers. It calms over-stressed adrenal glands and so helps prevent and relieve fatigue. Licorice root also contains phyto-estrogens that help to ease menopausal

symptoms. As a homeopathic remedy, sarsaparilla (wild licorice) is good for painful urination.

Licorice flower essence has a tranquilizing effect and calms restless, hyperactive behaviour; a good remedy for insomnia.

Ginkgo *or* Maidenhair Tree

LATIN NAME: *Ginkgo biloba*
FAMILY: *Ginkgoaceae*

"Ingest my timeless healing medicine and feel my life-enhancing energy enliven your whole being."

Most ancient of all medicinal plants, the dignified ginkgo tree comes from the age of the dinosaurs. The spirit of ginkgo has a revitalizing quality and inspires a desire to live forever.

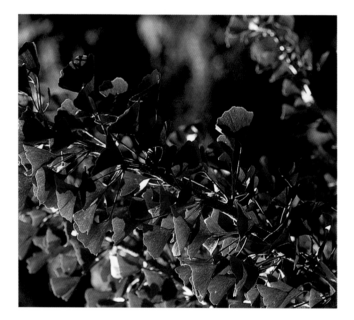

ABOVE *Ginkgo, growing as it has for millions of years, is venerated in the Far East.*

ORIGIN
The ginkgo tree is native to China and is central to Chinese medicine.

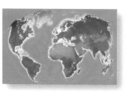

PLANT SPIRIT MEDICINES

Relish the enlivening spirit of ginkgo by eating its yellow plum-shaped fruits.

As a Chinese herbal medicine, ginkgo has long been seen as an elixir of youth that enhances and extends life. Science shows the leaves are rich in substances such as quercetin and catechin tannis, which increase blood supply and oxygenation of the tissues. As a herbal remedy, ginkgo shows promise as a smart drug for age-related memory loss.

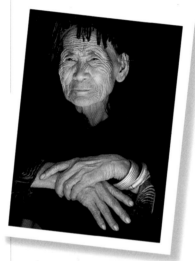

ABOVE *Ginkgo has always been associated with the secret of a long and healthy life.*

It may also help treat atherosclerosis, tinnitus, vertigo, and impotence.

SPIRIT AND SYMBOLISM

The last survivor of Mesozoic plants, which grew over 200 million years ago, ginkgo has lived through giant meteor strikes, mass extinctions, ice ages, nuclear explosions, and rising levels of pollution. Symbolizing endurance, resilience, and a determination to survive, a ginkgo tree may live to be a thousand years old.

Often growing to breathtaking heights, ginkgo bears fan-shaped leaves. Believed to be the oldest tree on the planet and considered sacred throughout the Far East, ginkgo trees have been cultivated in temple gardens and grounds for centuries. One of the most revered ginkgo trees, reputedly planted in the ninth century B.C.E., stands in the Buddhist monastery of Yongmun-san in Korea. Many make pilgrimages and say prayers to this amazing tree that reaches 180ft/55m into the sky. The ginkgo's life is interwoven with that of the people of Asia who have tapped into its amazing healing powers for over 5,000 years.

Sweet Grass *or* Seneca Grass

LATIN NAME: *Heirochloe odorata*

FAMILY: *Gramineae*

"My sweet smoke brings protection and takes your prayers and wishes to the heavens to be heard."

Sacred to the Native Americans, sweet grass is traditionally used in smudging ceremonies. Billows of sweet-smelling smoke cleanse the energies and carry sacred messages to the skies.

SPIRIT AND SYMBOLISM

In Native American legends, the fairies were so mesmerized by their own reflection in a pool that they pined away, leaving only the memory of their sweet scent lingering upon this green grass. When wind blows through the sweet grass as it grows on the plains of North America, you can almost hear their spirits whispering. The wisdom receiver of the Black Elk tribe says the spirit of Okaga, a good-hearted and generous being present in the wind that blows from the south, is carried in the smoke of sweet grass.

Waza, the chief of bad spirits who brings cold and death, runs from the spirit of Okaga and smudging with sweet grass will drive him away.

Sweet grass is used in almost all of the Black Elk's rituals. The leaves are cut and dried, then plaited to form braids that are lit and left to smolder.

RIGHT *Sweet grass can be found growing on the plains of North America and is revered by the Native Americans.*

ORIGIN
Sweet grass was originally found in North and South America.

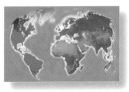

PLANT SPIRIT MEDICINES

As a sacred smoke, sweet grass is said to carry prayers to heaven. Native Americans believe that "Wakan Tanka," or nature, understands messages of smoke better than words. Used in ceremonies, sweet grass has

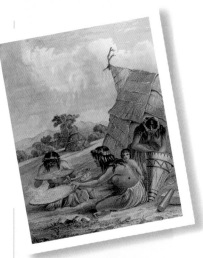

ABOVE *Californian women cleaning grass seed, from a sketch of 1856.*

purifying properties and encourages positive energies to be drawn to the sacred space. In Native American sweat lodge ceremonies, leaves are rubbed over the body as it sweats.

As a flower essence, sweet grass cleanses and revitalizes the etheric and physical bodies, sweeping away negative energies.

Sunflower

LATIN NAME: *Helianthus annuus*
FAMILY: *Compositae*

"I release all limitations and feel the warmth of the sun rising within me."

In every way the sunflower reflects the nature of its name. The broad-faced flowers gaze lovingly at the sun and follow its passage across the sky. The spirit of the sunflower brings lightness and warmth into the soul.

SPIRIT AND SYMBOLISM

Native to southwestern regions of North America, the sunflower was used by Incas and Aztecs as a symbol of the sun, whom they worshipped above all others. Vibrantly reaching skyward, the flowers show true devotion to the sun. In Greek mythology, Clytie, who adores the sun god Apollo, is turned into a sunflower. The sunflower has an honest, open, and sunny disposition. Its spirit helps the soul to harness the energy of the sun and dispel any darkness. It also absorbs pollutants from the air, making it cleaner for us to breathe.

ORIGIN
Sunflowers were originally discovered in the south-west states of North America.

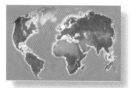

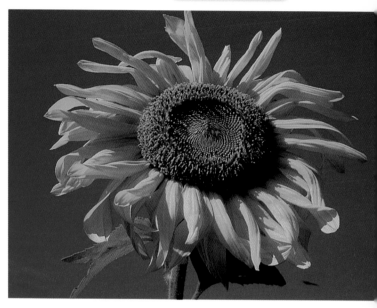

ABOVE *Everybody's favorite, the sunflower yields nourishing seeds, useful oil, and promotes good health.*

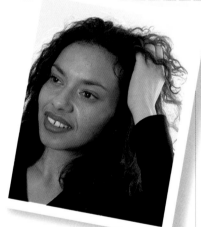

ABOVE *Give your hair a treat – condition with warm sunflower oil.*

PLANT SPIRIT MEDICINES

Sunflower seeds are a valuable source of nourishment. Rich in linoleic acid, they are recommended for weak eyes, fragile nails, and rough, dry skin. Roast them in soy sauce for a tasty snack.

Sunflower oil is good for stir-frying and dressings. It makes a useful oil for massage and a deep conditioning treatment for hair. Work some warm oil into the hair and scalp, then wrap in a warm damp towel and leave for **30 minutes** before shampooing.

As a flower essence, sunflower lights up our lives. It harmonizes the active masculine aspect of energy in both men and women, helps resolve conflicts with the father figure, and dissolves tensions from the past. The spirit of sunflower helps us become aware of who we are and brings an understanding of the correct role of ego.

Henbane

LATIN NAME: *Hyoscyamus niger*
FAMILY: *Solanaceae*

ORIGIN
Henbane was originally found across Europe.

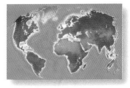

"With my visionary eyes, I can help you contact the spirit of loved ones."

A somewhat sinister looking plant, henbane has past associations with witchcraft. It opens the gateways to mystical worlds and brings the magical gift of flight.

SPIRIT AND SYMBOLISM

Commonly known as hog's bean, Jupiter's bean, and Devil's eye in Europe, henbane bears yellow flowers covered in dark purple veins that evoke an air of mystery and suspicion. Henbane's appearance alerts us to its poisonous nature, but its spirit holds the promise of magical journeys to enchanting worlds.

Henbane has hallucinatory and analgesic properties recognized since ancient times. It was an important medicine in the Mesopotamian pharmacopeia and Arabs still chew henbane to relieve stomach pains, seemingly immune to its dangers. The Roman historian Josephus implies that the head-dress of the ancient Jewish high priests was modelled on the flowers of this plant.

The Greek physician Dioscorides recognized henbane's pain-relieving qualities and the Romans may have introduced henbane to Britain. It was reputedly used in witches' potions to induce sensations of flying and turning into animals, which may have given rise to the popular idea of witches flying on broomsticks and becoming black cats.

LEFT *Henbane has sinister undertones, owing to its long association with witchcraft and magic potions.*

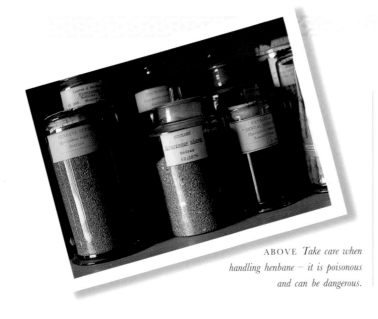

ABOVE *Take care when handling henbane – it is poisonous and can be dangerous.*

PLANT SPIRIT MEDICINES

The flowers and leaves yield hycosycamine and atropine, active principles similar to those found in belladonna; the whole plant is very poisonous. The potent narcotic and analgesic properties of henbane make it dangerous to use as a herbal remedy.

As a flower essence, henbane is perfectly safe and is a useful remedy for understanding death and exploring its realms or for those undergoing rites of passage. It aids connection with the spirits of the dead.

St. John's Wort

LATIN NAME: *Hypericum perforatum*
FAMILY: *Hypericaceae*

"I sweep away fears, inspire calm, and illuminate consciousness."

Like pockets of gold, St. John's Wort blooms on the fringes of woods and meadows, where its flowers can catch the sun's gentle rays. Despite its modest appearance, this plant is very versatile and heals on many different levels.

SPIRIT AND SYMBOLISM

The spirit of St. John's Wort has a subtly protective and uplifting nature. In fairy folklore it is the chief protective herb, healing illness due to bad spirits, essentially negative energies. Used in magic charms to safeguard the home from harm and loss, in Britain it was also taken to inspire lucid dreaming, a means of entering the dreaming world with awareness to gain subconscious insights.

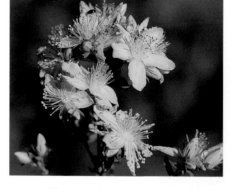

ABOVE *These attractive flowers produce lotions and creams to heal and soothe a plethora of ills.*

A fairy tale from the Isle of Wight says that if you tread on a piece of St. John's Wort on going to bed, the fairies will carry you through the night sky, taking you from place to place in a flight of fantasy. Its remedies lift the spirit from gloominess and help one to rise above any physical pain.

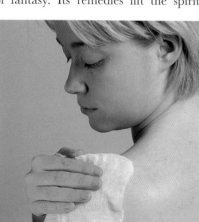

RIGHT *St. John's Wort is the ideal remedy for sunburn.*

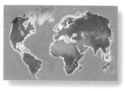

PLANT SPIRIT MEDICINES

St. John's Wort is the number one first-aid remedy. As a lotion, *Hypericum* cleanses and soothes skin wounds. Compresses soaked in this solution soothe burns, including sunburn, and reduce swellings. In creams, it is good for cuts, bites, burns, and bruises.

As a homeopathic remedy, *Hypericum* eases the shock of sudden painful injury. Infusions of leaves and flowers promote emotional balance, while stronger tinctures help to lift mild depression, including seasonal lows related to

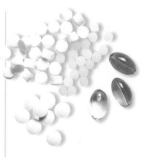

ABOVE *Homeopathic preparations of* Hypericum *help the shock of acute pain.*

sunlight deprivation. St. John's Wort flower essence relieves nervousness and fear by revitalizing the emotional subtle body. It promotes peaceful sleep and is a soothing remedy for childhood nightmares and hyperactivity.

LEFT *Use the essence of St. John's Wort to combat insomnia.*

Holly

LATIN NAME: *Ilex aquifolium*
FAMILY: *Aquifoliaceae*

"I help you to become a spiritual warrior using love as your source of power."

With its glossy leaves and scarlet berries, bushes of holly brighten the gloomy winter landscape. Long associated with Christmas festivities, holly helps to create an atmosphere of conviviality and an abundance of good cheer.

SPIRIT AND SYMBOLISM

Prickly leafed holly has a special place in the hearts of European folk. With its distinctly masculine spirit, holly may be envisaged as a sort of spiritual warrior who stimulates dynamic healing powers.

In folklore, holly is a lucky tree whose spirit acts as guardian to many fairies, elves, and pixies. Holly was sacred to the Druids, who brought it into their homes in winter to provide a haven for these fairy beings. In pagan times, holly water was sprinkled on newborns to keep them safe and happy.

In Roman times, holly was associated with the Saturnalia festival celebrated in mid-December and the Roman writer Pliny tells us that branches of holly protect houses from lightning and witchcraft, a notion that prevailed throughout medieval Europe. In Christianity, holly symbolizes the crown of thorns and the spirit of Christmas.

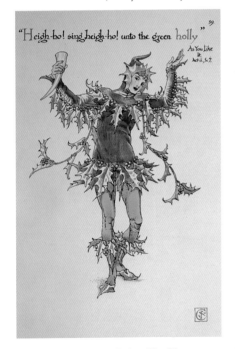

"Heigh-ho! sing heigh-ho! unto the green holly"

As You Like It. Act ii, S. 7.

ABOVE *Holly from* The Flower Fairies *by Walter Crane (1845–1915).*

ORIGIN
Holly is native to Europe.

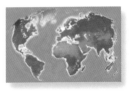

PLANT SPIRIT MEDICINES

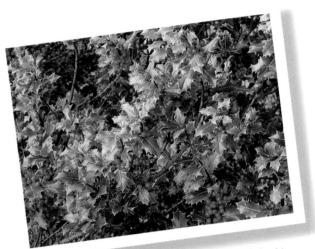

ABOVE *Festive and cheerful, beware the bright red berries of the holly.*

The berries of holly are poisonous, but the leaves have some therapeutic value. As an infusion, the dried leaves can be taken for chills and influenza. As a homeopathic remedy, holly is used as a substitute for quinine for intermittent fevers and eye problems. As a flower essence, holly is for when **we are enveloped in "prickly" or aggressive, emotions, such as anger, jealousy, bitterness, envy, rage, suspicion, revenge, hatred, bad temper, contempt, selfishness, and frustration.**

BELOW *Holly can provide a source of valuable cures for everyday complaints such as colds.*

Morning Glory

LATIN NAME: *Ipomoea violacea*
FAMILY NAME: *Convolvulaceae*

"With visionary powers, I empower and heal."

A jungle vine from South America with mesmerizing flowers in shades of sky blue, morning glory has visionary qualities. It enhances perception of the spirit world, restores faith in one's own spirituality, and brings freedom from destructive addictive habits.

SPIRIT AND SYMBOLISM

The spirit of morning glory is euphoric. Its amazing flowers open to greet the dawn and close as the sun sets. With a shape similar to satellites, they appear to draw in other spirit energies. Known to the Aztecs as oloiuhqui, morning glory was regarded as divine and used ceremonially for its visionary powers.

The Zapotec Indians of Oaxaca still use morning glory to help them contact the nature spirits, who yield visions of other jungle plants with healing powers.

ORIGIN
Morning glory originates from Central and South America.

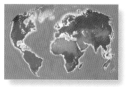

LEFT *The stunning morning glory plant is still revered in Central and South America, where it is used for its hallucinogenic properties.*

PLANT SPIRIT MEDICINES

Zapotec shamans grind morning glory seeds with a stone into a powder that is dissolved in water to make a visionary beverage. The seeds contain ergoline alkaloids chemically related to lysergic acid diethylamide, or LSD, which produce sensations of bright lights and color patterns. These feelings of euphoria give way to profound states of peace and relaxation. The seeds, however, are potentially toxic and should never be used by those unaware of their dangers.

The flower essence of morning glory enhances vitality and helps you to get up out of bed and greet the morning with enthusiasm, making it ideal for night owls with erratic sleeping habits. This essence helps to break addictive habits and brings freedom from dependency on drugs, such as opiates and nicotine opiates. At the same time it cleanses the body of associated side-effects of addiction. Morning glory restores faith in oneself and renews a belief in one's spiritual being.

Jasmine

LATIN NAME: *Jasminum officinalis*
FAMILY: *Oleaceae*

"My tiny delicate sensual flowers spiritualize human love."

Prized for its heavenly perfume, jasmine is a flower of sensuality and passionate love. Native to India, Persia, and China, this climbing plant with its starry flowers cascades over arbors in gardens throughout the world, filling them with its heady and luxurious scent.

SPIRIT AND SYMBOLISM

The spirit of jasmine is seductive. With her fine green tendrils, she weaves herself into one's affections and casts spells of love. She is a flower of fertility with a voluptuous and uplifting perfume that harmonizes all aspects of love.

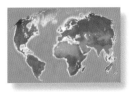

ORIGIN
Jasmine sums up the perfumes of its homelands of India, China, and Persia.

Throughout history, jasmine was linked to the moon goddess, and to ancient Egyptians she was often represented by Isis, who reputedly invented marriage. Held sacred in India, jasmine is known as the queen of the night since her perfume intensifies after sunset. Kama, the Hindu god of love, tipped his arrows of desire with jasmine blossom and the flowers are woven into Indian bridal wreaths. In China, jasmine is an emblem of beauty. Among Christians, the star-shaped blossoms portray heavenly fecundity.

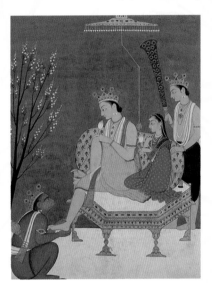

LEFT *The jasmine features in this painting of Hanuymen worshipping Rama, underlining its importance in Indian culture.*

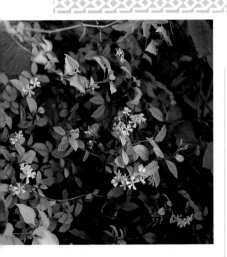

ABOVE *Vigorous and easy to grow, seductive jasmine is popular worldwide.*

PLANT SPIRIT MEDICINES

Jasmine is revered throughout the East as a perfume and medicine. In Indonesia, India, and China, women roll up jasmine blossoms into their newly washed and oiled hair before going to bed, and the perfume lingers for days.

In Indonesia, an infusion of *Jasminum sambac* flowers is used as an eye bath to treat infections. In China, jasmine flowers are blended with tea leaves to enrich the drink.

As a perfumed oil or absolute, jasmine enhances physical attraction and is a sexual tonic. Jasmine flower essence boosts sexual self-esteem and helps to transmute physical love into spiritual love. On a physical level it clears mucus congestion in the sinuses and lungs.

RIGHT *Beautiful container for a sensuous blossom.*

Juniper

LATIN NAME: *Juniperus communis*
FAMILY: *Cupressaceae*

"I restore the determination to succeed by overcoming life's obstacles of worry and defeatism."

A prickly evergreen shrub that grows wild on windswept moors and mountains, juniper has a robust and resolute nature. The spirit of juniper helps to clear away feelings of fear and failure.

SPIRIT AND SYMBOLISM

With its fresh, pine-like aroma and bittersweet berries, this hardy plant has been appreciated for centuries. Tibetans and Native Americans traditionally used juniper for spiritual purification. Sprigs were burned in ceremonial fires to create a clear, aromatic smoke which was thought to drive away negative energies and bad magic spells. Medicine men would waft juniper smoke around patients recovering from illness with sweeping movements, as if brushing the disease away. Fresh or dried leaves are tossed onto the hot rocks in the purifying sweat lodge ceremony. In Pueblo cultures, leaves are carried around in pouches and sewn into clothes, while Navajo women place a bracelet of juniper berries on babies and young children at bedtime to stop them having bad dreams.

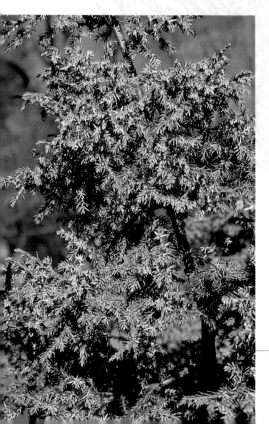

LEFT *The lush juniper plant has been used for hundreds of years for its healing properties and culinary benefits.*

ORIGIN
The juniper bush is a native of Europe.

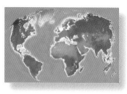

PLANT SPIRIT MEDICINES

Juniper wood and berries are burned on barbecues to impart their flavor and, like peppercorns, the berries can be crushed and used in cooking. Berries can be added to wines and liquors for their bittersweet taste and therapeutic properties. Gin, which owes its distinctive taste to juniper, was originally designed to be a diuretic medicine. As an infusion, juniper has warming and fortifying qualities. Essential oil of juniper benefits tiredness, cold hands and feet, fluid retention and lower backache. Add a few

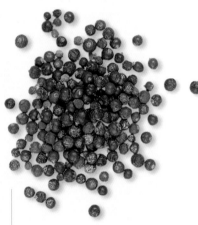

ABOVE *Flavorsome juniper berries enhance food and drinks.*

drops to a massage oil to ease aching joints and rheumatism. Burned as a vapor, it helps to clear feelings of stagnation. As a homeopathic remedy, juniper is indicated for kidney inflammation, edema, and disturbed digestion.

LEFT *Juniper is used in many remedies, such as cures for lethargy and indigestion.*

Bay Laurel

LATIN NAME: *Laurus nobilis*

FAMILY: *Lauraceae*

"I hold the vision of a belief in universal abundance and all possibilities."

This elegant small tree with its clusters of creamy-yellow flowers exudes an air of sophistication and accomplishment. The bay laurel's evergreen leaves symbolize success, while their warm qualities ward off wintertime ills.

SPIRIT AND SYMBOLISM

Bay laurel was revered by the ancient Greeks as a favorite of the gods, especially Apollo. According to myth, Apollo deemed the laurel garland a sign of success in artistic endeavors after the mountain nymph Daphne changed herself into a laurel tree to escape his amorous pursuits. At Delphi, site of Apollo's oracle, laurel was burned by temple priestesses as part of the prophetic ritual. Leaves were placed under a pillow at night to provoke prophetic dreams. The accomplished and victorious wore crowns of laurel leaves as a symbol of success and achievement. Asclepius, god of medicine, was always crowned with these magical leaves.

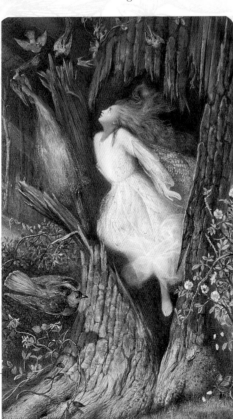

RIGHT The Metamorphosis of Daphne into a Laurel Tree by Apollo, *painted by Charles Sims (1873–1928).*

ORIGIN
Pungent bay leaves are native to Europe.

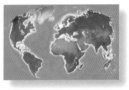

PLANT SPIRIT MEDICINES

RIGHT *Bay laurel leaves symbolise success: they also add flavor to foods and protect from disease.*

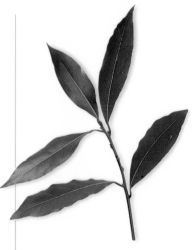

A protective plant said to keep away thunder, lightning, negativity, and disease, bay laurel was traditionally placed at the entrance of houses. The leaves have warming qualities that ward off winter ills such as colds, influenza, and coughs. Add them to vegetable broths, stocks, sauces, and stews.

Essential oil of bay laurel eases chronic bronchitis, influenza, rheumatic aches and pains. Add **10** drops of oil or a handful of fresh leaves to a hot bath. Its aroma uplifts the mind and aids concentration. Burn a few drops of oil when studying.

As a flower essence, bay laurel helps one to draw upon inner resources and manifest ideas. It's ideal for those who procrastinate and give up easily due to fear of taking risks.

LEFT *Oil and extract of bay laurel aid aches and pains, leaving one refreshed.*

Lavender

LATIN NAME: *Lavandula spp.*
FAMILY: *Labiatae*

"With my essence I refine and balance spiritual sensitivity, integrating it into daily life."

In sun-drenched Provence, shimmering fields of lavender color the landscape with a misty violet haze. Lavender has an air of cool purity that soothes and calms sensitive souls.

SPIRIT AND SYMBOLISM

With its silvery leaves and wispy flowers, the spirit of lavender combines sensitivity with stability. Growing wild around the Mediterranean, lavender prefers the mountains where the air is pure and clean.

Known in folklore as elf leaf and rabbit

ORIGIN
Lavender originates from Southern Europe.

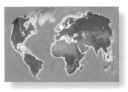

tobacco, lavender has been valued for it refreshing perfume and medicinal qualities since ancient times. The Greeks burned lavender as an incense offering and the Romans added sprigs to their bath water; in Latin, *lavare* means to wash.

Ancient Druids carried lavender to help them to see spirits and ward off evil influences. In magical midsummer ceremonies they tossed it onto bonfires as an offering to the gods and goddesses of nature.

LEFT *A carpet of purple transforms a landscape.*

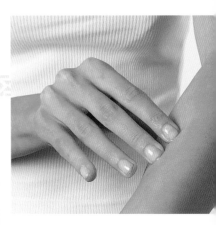

ABOVE *Lavender oil aids a variety of skin complaints and promotes quick healing.*

PLANT SPIRIT MEDICINES

As an infusion or tisane, lavender aids digestion and acts as a morning pick-me-up. At the first sign of a cold or influenza, gargle with lavender tea.

Lavender essential oil is the first choice for burns, cuts, and bruises. Dab a few drops of neat oil onto damaged skin to ease the pain and hasten healing. Use it in massage oils and creams for nervous skin conditions, such as eczema and psoriasis. Place a few drops on your pillow case to relieve insomnia. Stroke over your temples to ease tension headaches. As a floral water, lavender clarifies the skin and adds luster to hair.

Encapsulated in the flower essence, the spirit of lavender soothes nervous over-sensitivity, cleanses the meridians, and activates the crown chakra, so aiding fuller connection with the higher self.

Osha

LATIN NAME: *Ligisticum porteri*
FAMILY: *Umbelliferae*

"I am the sacred medicine gift that draws in powerful healing."

Known to Native Americans as bear medicine, the spirit of osha is strong and warrior-like. Bears go to great lengths to find these root, which promise potent remedies for some of our commonest ills.

SPIRIT AND SYMBOLISM

Like a bear curled up in its den, osha's potency lies in its hairy root. Osha is a wild plant that defies domestication. It lives in the mountains and alpine clearings of Mexico, New Mexico, and Colorado.

ORIGIN
The osha root can be found in America and Mexico.

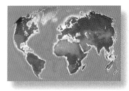

With its strength of spirit, osha exudes bear energy. The tribal warriors carried the osha root as a talisman, while elders have always regarded osha as a gift of medicine revealed in visions by the spirit of the bear. To healers and medicine men osha is sacred and revered for its healing powers.

Bears love osha. On emerging from hibernation, a bear will dig up the root and chew it to form a watery paste, which it uses to wash its face. Males dig up roots and offer them to females as part of courtship.

LEFT *Native North Americans believe that the spirit of the bear holds the secrets of plant medicine.*

PLANT SPIRIT MEDICINES

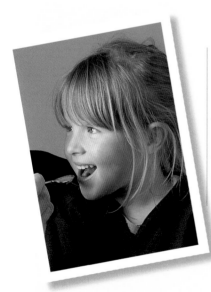

LEFT *Soothing osha helps alleviate colds and sore throats.*

Osha is a protective medicine with potent antiviral properties. Prepared as a decoction, osha tea should be sipped at the first sign of flu and colds to minimize symptoms. Apaches also drink osha tea to relieve indigestion and stomach cramps. Syrups containing osha are excellent for sore throats and bronchial infections. As a tincture, osha can be used for bathing skin cuts and wounds to prevent any kind of infection.

Imbibing the spirit of osha helps those struggling with their own inner demons to face the darkness inside their soul. It is a good herb to have in your sacred medicine bundle, but be prepared – osha heightens emotions and fuels passions.

Apple

LATIN NAME: *Malus spp.*

FAMILY: *Rosaceae*

"I help to unlock the true wellspring of health and bring harmony to life."

With pastel pink blossoms that turn into rose-blushed fruits, the apple is the tree of enchantment. The spirit of the apple holds the knowledge of eternal youth and beauty.

SPIRIT AND SYMBOLISM

The bearer of life-giving fruit, apples have always had a sacred significance. Symbolizing love, happiness, and fertility, the apple was once seen as a magical fruit, synonymous with paradise. In Greek mythology Gaia, the earth goddess, made a gift of the golden apples of Hesperides to Hera on her marriage to Zeus, and one of Heracle's labors was to gather these precious fruits.

In British legend, King Arthur disappeared to the Isles of Apples, or Avalon, the name given to paradise or fairyland, and Lancelot was sleeping under an apple tree when he was carried away by the four fairy queens.

In fairy traditions, the spirit of apple takes on the form of a beautiful woman who opens the heart to new love; her flower fairies bring gifts of happiness, love, and healing. The apple tree was home to the mythical unicorn, who lived beneath its blossom-drenched branches.

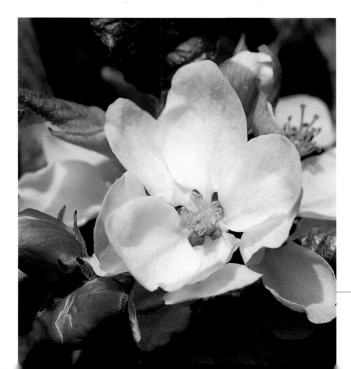

ORIGIN

Apples come from Europe.

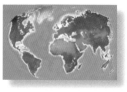

PLANT SPIRIT MEDICINES

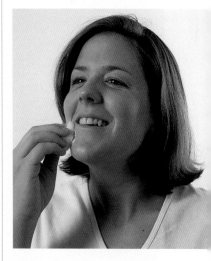

ABOVE *Bite into the tasty fruit and release the detoxifying agents which aid digestion.*

Brimming with goodness, apples also have remarkable cleansing properties, clarifying the complexion, refreshing and toning the gums, while removing toxins from the digestive system. A little raw grated apple helps to clear diarrhea, while stewed apple is good for constipation. An apple tea made from dried apple slices

LEFT *The delicate blossom of the apple tree can be used as an extract to enhance well-being.*

cleanses the urinary tract. As a beauty tonic, cider vinegar diluted with water restores the natural pH balance of hair, scalp, and skin. As a flower essence, apple blossom detoxifies the mind and body to restore emotional well-being. It also draws in spiritual energies and is known to encourage a healthy outlook on life.

ABOVE *Cider vinegar applied to the skin refreshes and tones.*

Mandrake

LATIN NAME: *Mandragora officinarum*
FAMILY: *Solanaceae*

"My sacred ingredients will help you to enter the magical dream-time and contact the power within."

Mandrake is a mystical plant seen since ancient times as a symbol of enchantment, fertility, and prosperity. The spirit of the mandrake dispels illusions, attracts love, and allows us to realize the soul is everlasting.

SPIRIT AND SYMBOLISM

Ancient Egyptian tomb decorations and papyri show how highly esteemed mandrake was and how it may have been used for astral or spiritual journeys. The flowers, leaves, and green fruits, like unripe tomatoes, all have extraordinary powers.

A fourteenth century B.C bas-relief shows the Egyptian healer queen, Meriton, offering her consort Semenkhara two mandrakes and a blue water lily. A chest from Tutankhamun's tomb depicts his wife offering the ailing king narcotic blue lilies and opium poppy fruits; she wears mandrake fruits on her head and two servants are picking mandrakes for the couple. It is said the high priests used mandrake and blue lily to enter a deep trance or "little death" in which the spirit left the physical body to communicate with beings on other planes.

In medieval times, many people esteemed mandrake for its pain-killing properties and it was regarded as a cure for impotence and sterility.

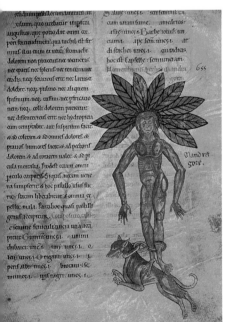

LEFT *The root of the mandrake is portrayed in human form in this 12th-century illuminated medical treatise.*

ORIGIN
The mandrake is a native of Egypt.

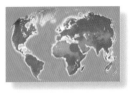

PLANT SPIRIT MEDICINES

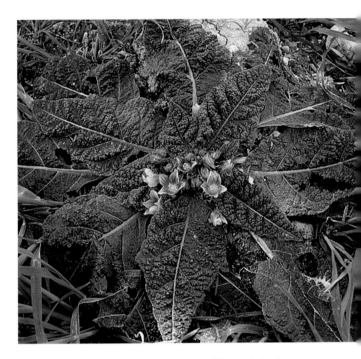

Mandrake roots and fruits contain the powerful relaxant drug hyoscine, used in medicine as a pre-anesthetic. The plant is quite poisonous and should never be prepared for personal use at home.

Mandragora is used as a homeopathic remedy to treat restless excitability,

ABOVE *The mandrake plant should be treated with respect; its properties are very powerful.*

body weakness, and overwhelming desires to sleep. As a flower essence, mandrake connects a person to that which is eternal within and builds confidence by overcoming the illusion of powerlessness.

Mango

LATIN NAME: *Mangifera indica*
FAMILY: *Anacardiaceae*

*"With sensuous and heavenly fruit of the Gods,
I bring spiritual nourishment."*

The flower and fruits of the mango appear to be heaven-sent. Sprays of white star-shaped blossoms perfume tropical air with a richly sensuous scent. With their velvety smooth succulent golden flesh, these fruits belong to paradise.

SPIRIT AND SYMBOLISM

Originating in the foothills of the Himalayas, the mango was honored as a fruit of the gods throughout Asia. The tree prefers to grow high above sea level where the air is pure and clear. The cultivation of mangoes began some 4,000 years ago. Even the most poetic descriptions of this fruit cannot do it justice. It has long played an important role in Hindu culture and religion, where traditionally, mangoes are known as "fruits of heavenly joy." We now know they contain two compounds, anacardic acid and ancardiol, which are closely related chemically to some antidepressant drugs.

ORIGIN
*Mangoes came from
India and Burma.*

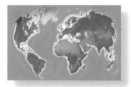

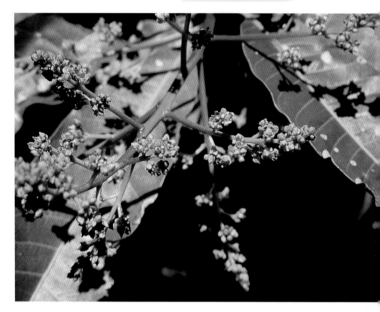

ABOVE *The mango flower essence
encourages spiritual nourishment and growth.*

PLANT SPIRIT MEDICINES

There are many ways to savor these lush fruits. Peel back the skin and enjoy the succulent flesh as nature intended. Rich in vitamin C and carotenes, mangoes provide nutritious properties and soothe the digestive system.

LEFT *Tempting slices of
mango contain beneficial
nutrients to aid digestion.*

As a herbal preparation, the bark of mango tree is used by medicine men in the Pacific islands to treat various ills. In homeopathic doses, mango is used by professionals to stop bleeding, especially uterine bleeding.

As a flower essence, mango increases one's ability to assimilate the higher frequencies of cosmic energy which assist spiritual growth and reduce the need for denser physical foods such as meat.

Tea Tree

LATIN NAME: *Melaleuca alternifolia*
FAMILY: *Myrtaceae*

"I help the physically delicate to gain strength and empowerment."

Found only in Australia, tea tree has been used as a medicine by native Aborigines for generations. By bolstering the body's resilience, this spindly shrub, with its yellow-green, bottle-brush flowers, treats a broad spectrum of ills.

SPIRIT AND SYMBOLISM

A cousin to eucalyptus, tea tree belongs to a close-knit family of paperbark trees noted for their strong medicinal scent. The spirit of the tea tree is strong and assertive, with its roots firmly planted on the ground, favoring swampy coastal regions. The Aborigines use it to make small canoes, knife sheaths, and thatches for shelters, as well as chewing and brewing the leaves to make medicine for treating coughs, colds, and headaches.

In a therapy handed down through generations, the Bundjalung Aborigines crush the leaves and combine them with mud to make a pack for treating infections and a wide range of skin conditions.

ORIGIN
The healing tea tree originates from Australia.

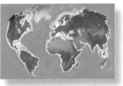

LEFT *The versatile tea tree is an integral part in the life of the Aborigine people.*

BELOW The Heart Chakra, *1927, demonstrating the tea tree's spiritual qualities.*

PLANT SPIRIT MEDICINES

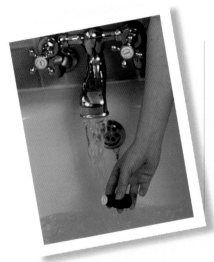

LEFT *Oil of the tea tree added to your bath helps stop infection.*

Tea tree is now known to be a potent antiseptic and is an excellent first-aid remedy. An infusion of tea tree leaves makes a good mouthwash, skin splash for acne-prone complexions, and hair rinse for keeping head-lice in children at bay. Adding **8-10** drops of tea tree essential oil to the bath twice a week boosts resistance to all forms of infection. Diluted in water, it can be used as a disinfectant for spraying rooms.

As a flower essence, tea tree opens the heart chakra while clearing and rebalancing energy in all the meridians.

Mint

LATIN NAME: *Mentha spp.*
FAMILY: *Labiatae*

"I am a visionary spirit, a herb of inspiration, clear insight, and dreams of prophecy."

Cool and refreshing, mint is admired throughout the world. Since the earliest times its bright and inspiring qualities have been used to clear the mind and bring flashes of insight.

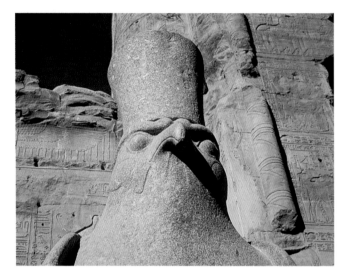

ABOVE *The Falcon of Horus in the court of the Temple of Horus at Edfu, c. 332–30 B.C.E.*

SPIRIT AND SYMBOLISM

The spirit of mint is as clear as crystal and for this reason this plant was once used as a visionary tool to enhance intuition and bring spiritual insights.

The ancient Egyptians recognized mint's powers, dedicating it to their sun god Horus and using it as a ritual perfume as well as an ingredient of their sacred "kyphi." In Greek mythology, mint sprang from the seductive nymph, Minthe, who is discovered by Persephone in the arms of her husband Hades. In a fit of jealousy, Persephone crushes her, but Hades gave her new life as a plant. In ancient Greece and Rome, mint was used to scent baths and bedding, its aroma being a familiar part of daily life.

ORIGIN
The domestic mint plant was originally found growing in Africa.

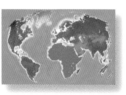

PLANT SPIRIT MEDICINES

In cooking, mint refreshes the taste buds and aids digestion. An infusion of mint improves circulation and promotes sweating, which reduces a fever. In hot climates mint has a cooling effect. Mint tea is wonderfully digestive and also quells feelings of nausea and sickness.

As a compress, mint eases pain and relieves bruising and swelling. Essential oil of mint clears the mind, promotes concentration, and alleviates mental fatigue. If applying to the body it must always be diluted.

Peppermint flower essence is for spiritual trials and tribulations when one feels overwhelmed and full of despair. It brings calmness and a readiness to embrace new beginnings.

LEFT *An infusion of mint creates a delicious tea to settle the stomach.*

Myrtle

LATIN NAME: *Myrtus communis*
FAMILY: *Myrtaceae*

"I offer protection by inspiring enduring love."

In days past fragrant myrtle flowers were found in every bride's bouquet. The spirit of this flower inspires and perpetuates love. Grown throughout the Mediterranean, myrtle is a symbol of lasting happiness and good fortune.

ORIGIN
Myrtle was first found in Africa.

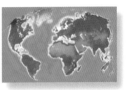

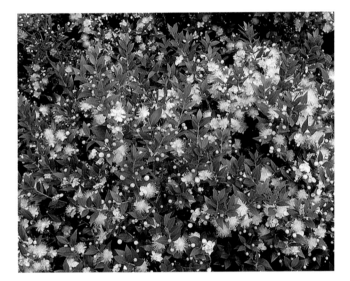

ABOVE *In full blossom the myrtle displays a beauty revered by the Ancient Greeks.*

SPIRIT AND SYMBOLISM

Myrtle might be mistaken for any evergreen shrub until, bedecked with sprays of white blossom, she takes on a bridal beauty. Myrtle is regarded as an embodiment of love and since earliest times has been used in marriage ceremonies. To the ancient Greeks, she was the incarnation of Aphrodite, the divine goddess of love.

In Rome, Venus was worshipped under the name of Myrtea in her temple at the foot of the Aventine. Here branches of myrtle were an essential accompaniment to all religious ceremonies. In the South of France, a myrtle tree planted near the house is thought to offer protection from the evil eye, but it has to be planted by a woman.

PLANT SPIRIT MEDICINES

The ancient Egyptians recognized the therapeutic power of myrtle and steeped the leaves in wine to counter fever and infection. In France myrtle is used to make popular liquor drinks with similar protective properties.

The dark green leaves contain vesicles full of camphory essential oils. These make good cleansers for oily complexions and skin that is prone to acne. Make a refreshing skin-cleansing lotion using 3½ tablespoons/50ml rosewater and 5 drops of myrtle oil.

The clean, camphory aroma of myrtle clears and protects the respiratory system, as well as keeping insects at bay. Plant a bush near your house to ward off mosquitoes.

As a flower essence, myrtle helps to project the healing energy of love over long distances.

RIGHT *As oils and infusions, the myrtle protects and cleanses the body both inside and out.*

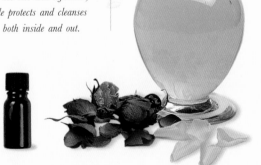

Lotus

LATIN NAME: *Nelumbo nucifera*
FAMILY: *Nymphaeaceae*

"I am the king of the flowers and my gift is spiritual enlightenment."

The most spiritual of all flowers, lotus is an embodiment of purity and perfection. Rising out of the mud and water, this immaculate flower represents our potential and aspirations for spiritual enlightenment.

THE SPIRIT OF THE LOTUS

Considered sacred throughout the Middle and Far East, and by the Aborigines of northern Australia, the lotus is said to be the first flower on earth. Its spirit is pure and holds the wisdom of the world. Breathtaking white, pink, or red flowers are carried on elegant stems representing the umbilical cord that binds man to his origins. Petals open at dawn and close at sunset, suggesting the cycle of birth and rebirth.

ORIGIN
Lotus is native to Egypt, Central Asia, India, and China.

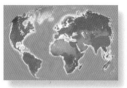

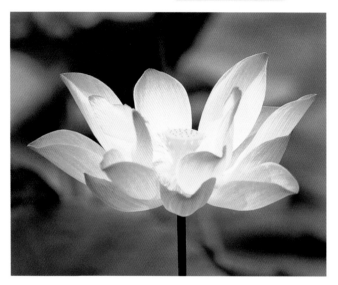

ABOVE *Beauty unfolded – the lotus flower symbolises flawlessness and sagacity.*

SYMBOLISM

In Hindu mythology, the lotus of a thousand petals represents the sun emerging from the cosmic ocean and symbolizes divine birth for the creative god Brahma, who emerges from a golden lotus. In Buddhism, the Buddha is often represented as a jewel seated on a lotus. In the Lotus Sutra, Buddha tells that teaching and

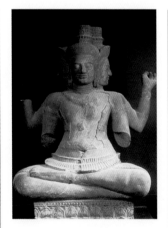

ABOVE *Sculpture of Brahma from Batambang, Cambodia, mid 10th century.*

perfecting wisdom is the only vehicle to salvation.

Ancient Egyptians believed the lotus was the first living thing to appear on earth. Its petals unfurled to reveal the supreme God, representing intellectual rulership. Capitals of Egyptian columns were carved as lotuses, in bud and full flower, and fresh flowers were

presented as offerings to the gods.

In Greek mythology, Lotis, Poseidon beautiful daughter was transformed into a lotus tree to safeguard her from amorous Priapus, the personification of male sexual power. Homer tells that anyone who ate her fruits lost all sense of reality, forgetting all troubles and cares.

Lotus

ESSENCE OF SPIRITUAL ENLIGHTENMENT

The spirit of lotus is encapsulated in its flower essence.

• A spiritual elixir and master healer that encourages receptivity and openness.

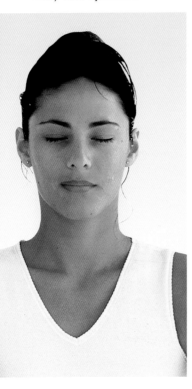

• It opens the crown chakra to higher energies while balancing and aligning all the chakras.

• Known for cleansing and strengthening the aura, it also clears the entire system of toxins.

• It harmonizes interpersonal relationships and purifies the emotions.

• Lotus flower essence calms the mind and improves concentration. It is also useful in meditation.

LEFT *Meditating in the Lotus position clears the mind and maintains the body's balance.*

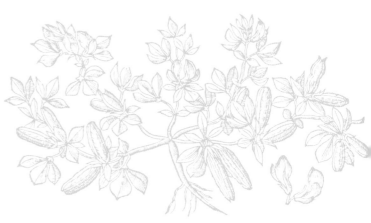

ABOVE *Depicted in art throughout the ages, the lotus is instantly recognizable.*

• It amplifies the effect of other remedies, particularly other flower essences.

Cultivated in China as a food and medicine for at least 3,000 years, lotus is rich in vitamins B, C, and E. The roots of the lotus plant may be roasted, pickled, candied, or sliced and even served as fries. Medicinally the fruits, seeds, and roots are used to arrest bleeding and for treating problems of the heart, kidneys, and spleen.

PLANT SPIRIT MEDICINES

To stop nosebleeds, drink the juice of a few freshly squeezed lotus roots. *Lotus plumule*, the green bud of a ripe lotus seed, is used as a heart tonic and appears

to lower bloo
pressure. But
as an incense
perfume of l
reminds us o
inner sanctit
and divinity.

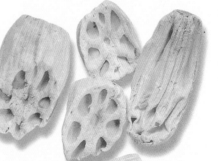

LEFT *Roots of the lotus contain properties which alleviate internal ailments; they also make tasty snacks.*

Tobacco

LATIN NAME: *Nicotiana tabacum*
FAMILY: *Solanaceae*

"My sacred smoke calms a restless spirit and aids in communication with the ancestral grandfathers."

Traditionally used as a sacred offering, tobacco was once seen as a magical and medicinal herb. Used in sacred ceremonies and rituals, the smoke from the tobacco leaves enhances our perception and appreciation of the spirit world.

SPIRIT AND SYMBOLISM

The spirit of tobacco has a peaceful and exhilarating quality. This has long been known to Native Americans, who have always used tobacco leaves as a sacred offering and smoke them in their pipes of peace.

Tobacco was used by healer priests in sacred ceremonies throughout the ancient Americas. Today, Campa Indians of the Peruvian rainforest combine tobacco and ayahuasca as a shamanic sacrament in nocturnal rituals to alter states of consciousness. The Warao Indian shamans in Venezuela smoke large cigars of local tobacco to enter a narcotic trance in which they commune with supreme spirits, or kanobos, dwelling in the mountains.

Tobacco was first planted in Europe as a strange and marvelous medicinal herb for curing anything from animal and insect bites to headaches, colds, bruises, asthma, and giddiness.

RIGHT Not only for smoking, tobacco is a versatile plant used in the treatment of many ills as well as in ritual practices.

ORIGIN
The tobacco plant was found growing in Peru and Ecuador.

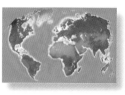

PLANT SPIRIT MEDICINES

The leaves of tobacco can be used as an offering in a sacred ceremony of thankfulness. In Chinese medicine, pure, unadulterated tobacco is seen as warm and pungent. It promotes energy circulation and is recommended for indigestion, headache, abdominal swelling, and the pain from arthritis. As a homeopathic remedy, *Nicotiana tabacum* is indicated for alleviating the nausea of motion sickness that is better after breathing fresh air.

As a flower essence, tobacco clears the effects of nicotine from the body, dissolving dependency and addition to cigarettes. It helps to rebalance and calm the whole body system.

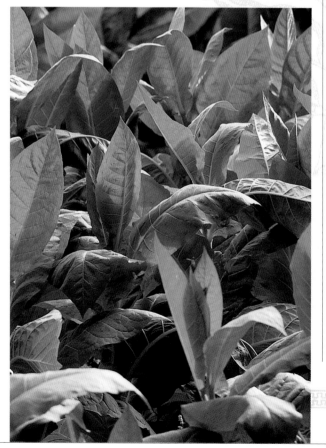

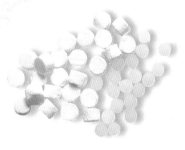

ABOVE Extract of tobacco can calm and even aid in dispelling nicotine addiction.

Water Lily *and* Blue Water Lily

LATIN NAMES: *Nymphaea alba and N. caerulea*
FAMILY: *Nymphaeaceae*

"With my sensual flower I embody tranquility and the purity of unconditional love. I am the essence of a soul seeker."

Appearing like an apparition upon the water, water lilies have an unearthly quality. Floating so serenely, this flower evokes a sense of divine peace and innocence.

SPIRIT AND SYMBOLISM

With cup-shaped flowers like hands open to receive a spiritual blessing, the spirit of water lily inspires purity, virtue, intimacy, and unconditional love. From the stunning, tropical magenta water lilies that bloom only during the night to the delicate pink and white blossoms adorning the Kashmir lakes at the foot of the snow-clad Himalayan mountains, water lilies hold one spellbound by their beauty. Like perfumed mist, their sweet scent hangs in the air.

Nyphmaea is derived from the Greek for water-nymph and virgin. German peasants believed that water nymphs disguised themselves as water lilies when pestered by lustful males. In the Middle Ages, a maiden carrying water lilies was able to resist the magical influence of love potions. The blue water lily is the sensuous cousin. It was sacred to the ancient Egyptians, who may have used it to heighten sexual pleasure. It is depicted on the walls of King Tutankhamun's tomb with other narcotic plants and appears to have evoked a sense of euphoric tranquility and heightened awareness in which perceptions are altered. The blue water lily appears to have embodied many of the virtues of their sacred lotus.

ORIGIN
The water lily was discovered in Asia.

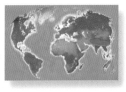

PLANT SPIRIT MEDICINES

As a perfume, water lily seduces the senses and kindles feelings of unearthly desire. As a flower essence, water lily is the Kama Sutra of flower extracts. A powerful tonic for those with psychological inhibitions about intimacy and sex, it heightens sensuality and enhances enjoyment of love-making. Use it for fostering unconditional love in a relationship.

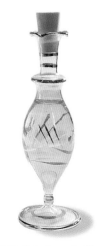

ABOVE *Seductive water lily perfume has a long history.*

BELOW *Gently floating on the water, the beautiful water lily is associated with myth and sensuality.*

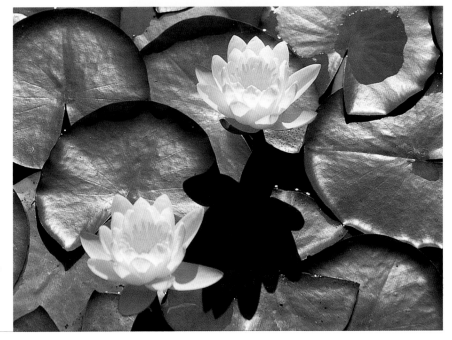

Basil *or* Sweet Basil

ORIGIN
The basil plant is native to India.

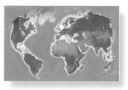

LATIN NAME: *Ocimum basilicum*
FAMILY: *Labiatae*

"I help to harmonize spirituality and sexuality."

Often associated with the sunny Mediterranean, sweet-smelling basil's true home is India, where it is considered sacred. This fresh green herb reminds us that true pleasure springs from the union of the physical and the spiritual.

SPIRIT AND SYMBOLISM

Basil is a protective plant whose purpose is to integrate spirituality with physical desire. Known as holy basil, or tulsi, in Hindu religion it is

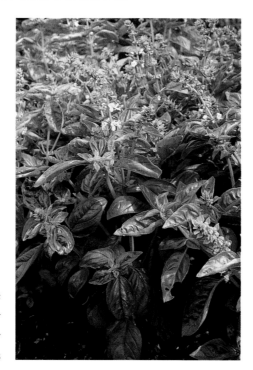

LEFT *Prolific basil has been associated with many religions across the world.*

pervaded with the divinity of Vishnu, who embodies love, truth, order, and mercy. Pots of basil adorn Hindu temples, where its aroma opens the heavens to the worshipper.

Cultivated in the Middle East since ancient times, Jews traditionally hold sprays of basil to give them strength during religious fasts. Arabs consider its scent to be a potent aphrodisiac.

Druids saw basil as a magical and protective herb that restored love and friendship in quarreling couples. It was used in love spells and sprinkled over a loved one while asleep to ensure fidelity.

PLANT SPIRIT MEDICINES

As a culinary herb basil has a refreshing flavor and makes dishes easier to digest. To ensure a constant fresh supply and drive mosquitoes away, grow pots of basil on the windowsill.

An infusion of basil tea helps to relieve headaches and migraine, diarrhea, stomach aches, and menstrual pains. Essential oil of basil makes a good massage oil for fortifying the

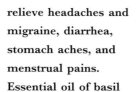

LEFT *Rub in oil of basil to promote a relaxed mind and body.*

nervous system, relieving stress, and soothing anxiety.

Basil flower essence is for those who see sexuality and spirituality as separate and helps bring the two together. It eliminates such conflicts and integrates spiritual bliss with physical pleasure.

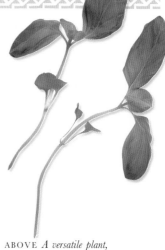

ABOVE *A versatile plant, basil improves flavor and aids digestion.*

Evening Primrose

LATIN NAME: *Oenothera biennis*

FAMILY: *Onagraceae*

"I bring lightness and warmth to the inner child and nourishment to women."

This delicate flower encapsulates the golden glow of the sun as it sets below the horizon. Its spirit is warming and reassuring. Evening primrose nourishes on many levels and in so doing brings relief from a spectrum of health problems.

SPIRIT AND SYMBOLISM

Named for its bright yellow flowers that open in the early evening, this tall biennial herb was highly valued by the Native Americans. Its spirit warms and lightens every corner of our being. The native Indians soaked the whole plant in warm water to make poultices for healing bruises and wounds and soothing inflamed skin. They also ate the tiny seeds to aid recovery from infections.

ORIGIN

Evening primrose originates from North America.

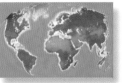

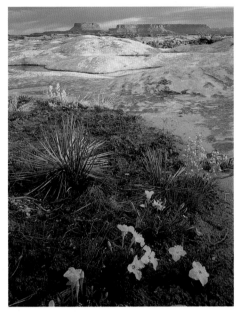

LEFT *Growing here in the arid Utah landscape, the evening primrose provides a welcome splash of color. Prized by Native Americans, it is recognized as a valuable medicine throughout the world.*

PLANT SPIRIT MEDICINES

The oil derived from evening primrose seeds is rich in gamma linolenic acid, or GLA, a substance found in the membranes surrounding every cell in the body. It is also made into prostaglandins, hormone-like substances that regulate many bodily

ABOVE

Capsules of oil of primrose give relief to a wide range of ills.

processes. For this reason, evening primrose oil can help treat many health problems ranging from premenstrual tension

to mood swings, alcohol addiction, and obesity, along with skin problems such as eczema and acne.

Rub evening primrose oil directly onto the skin, which will gladly soak up the GLA. Add a little to your favorite skin-care cream and massage into any rough or dehydrated areas. As a dietary supplement,

take a 250mg tablet of evening primrose oil at least twice a day.

As a flower essence, the spirit of evening primrose balances female cycles, which can often become upset by feelings of sexual and emotional repression. It brings emotional warmth and the ability to form committed relationships.

Olive

LATIN NAME: *Olea europaea*
FAMILY: *Oleaceae*

"I offer you the hand of peace and tranquility."

Olive trees have adorned the Aegean islands since the dawn of time. With their silvery leaves shimmering beneath the crystal clear skies, these ancient trees evoke a sense of timelessness and divine peace.

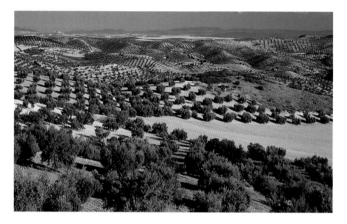

ABOVE *Olive groves in Andalusia, Spain, as they have been for centuries across southern Europe.*

SPIRIT AND SYMBOLISM

Since early times, the olive has been regarded as sacred. When Noah's dove returned to the Ark after the rains had ceased, it bore an olive twig, a sign sent by God to indicate peace and reconciliation. The ancient Greeks worshipped the olive as Athena, the goddess of wisdom and learning. For the men of Attica, fruits from the olive tree were considered divine and from the era of Pericles onwards, the coins of Athens were stamped with an olive branch. In Judaism, olive oil is considered holy and is used as fuel for the Sabbath lamp and for the menorah in the festival of Hanukkah.

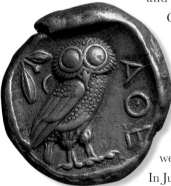

ABOVE *Athena coin, c. 440 B.C.E., depicts the wise owl and the olive branch.*

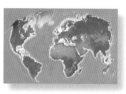

PLANT SPIRIT MEDICINES

RIGHT *Revitalize your hair with a treatment of warm olive oil to add shine.*

Olives and their oil are one of the richest sources of vitamin E, along with other essential nutrients. Cold-pressed olives produce the best quality virgin oil. To reap its goodness, sprinkle olive oil onto leafy salads and use it in cooking. Being rich in monounsaturated fatty acids, it appears to exert a protective influence on the heart and circulatory system.

In France, doctors recommend olives for diabetes and liver trouble, while in Chinese medicine sucking an olive is said to relieve sore throats. Used as a beauty treatment, olive oil softens skin and restores luster to dull hair. A little warm

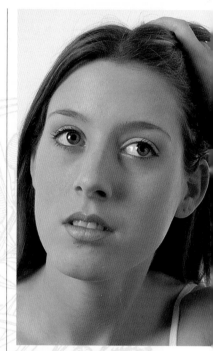

oil works wonders for clearing cradle cap in babies.

Olive flower essence can uplift those suffering from mental and physical exhaustion. Like a Greek island holiday, the spirit of olive recuperates the spirit and combats the effects of overwork and worry.

Orchid

LATIN NAME: *Orchis*
FAMILY: *Orchidaceae*

"I am the connection between man, the earth, and the cosmos; my task is to accelerate man's spiritual evolution."

These delicate flowers with their wing-shaped petals resemble tiny angelic beings. If flower fairies were to materialize, they would surely take the form of these ethereal-looking flowers.

ORIGIN
The orchid is native to both the Amazon and Australia.

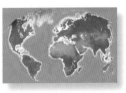

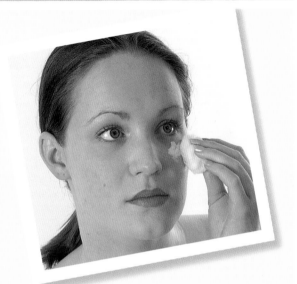

ABOVE *Good for the face, orchid oil moisturizes dry or aging skin.*

SPIRIT AND SYMBOLISM

The spirit of the orchid is angelic. It shows us how delicate and beautiful earthly forms can be. Attuning to the spirit of orchids is said to accelerate one's spiritual evolution and help to connect us with the devas and angels and perhaps even reach their higher spiritual plane.

The orchid family contains many species, too numerous to mention, but wonderfully rich in their variety. Orchids are some of the youngest species in the plant kingdom, having evolved relatively recently.

The orchids of Europe

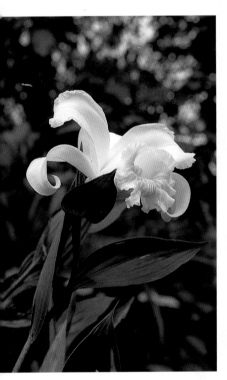

ABOVE *An orchid from the rainforest of Costa Rica, one of many stunning varieties across the world.*

and the Mediterranean are deeply rooted in the earth, while the orchids of the Amazon rainforests are found growing 35ft/10.7m up in the tree tops. The roots of these heaven-bound orchids have seemingly lost contact with the earth. The jungle shamans believe these orchids enjoy close contact with the spirit world and can help those who come to them for their properties to try and contact this world.

PLANT SPIRIT MEDICINES

The oil extracted from orchids is valued for its therapeutic, healing, and soothing properties. It helps to replenish skin cells with moisture and as such is a prized ingredient of creams for dehydrated skin.

As a flower essence, the orchid can aid the spiritual evolution of mankind. It helps to reconnect us with the spirit world by acting as a messenger between the earthly and the spiritual planes. The spirit energy of the orchid vibrates at a very high frequency that resonates with those of our own higher chakras and subtle bodies, so refining our powers of perception.

Marjoram

LATIN NAME: *Origanum spp.*
FAMILY: *Labiatae*

"I restore your ability to trust in life's protecting and preserving force."

There is perhaps no herb that evokes a sense of the Mediterranean as abundantly as marjoram. In Greek, its name means "joy of the mountains," reflecting the uplifting yet reassuring nature of this well-loved little plant.

SPIRIT AND SYMBOLISM

Growing wild in sunny Mediterranean climes, marjoram has a strong spirit that brings warmth and comfort. It reminds us that life never ends, but begins another cycle. In Hinduism, marjoram is sacred to Vishnu, the preserver of the universe, and to Shiva, the mountain god who performs the great dance of creation and destruction.

Cultivated by the ancient Egyptians, pot marjoram (*Origanum onites*) was dedicated to Osiris, the eternally dying and rising god who was king of the afterlife. In Greece,

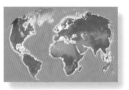

ORIGIN
Marjoram is a native of southern Europe.

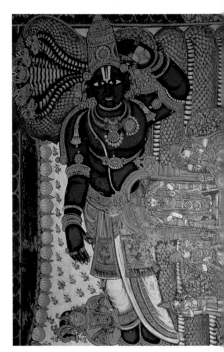

marjoram is a herb of happiness; young married couples are crowned with the flowers as a symbol of love and honor and it is also placed on graves to bring joy and spiritual peace to the deceased. In European folklore, marjoram is used to create love spells and potions to banish depression.

RIGHT *Wall painting of the God Vishna from Shree Rangan Temple, Trichi, India. Note the marjoram pattern on the carpet.*

PLANT SPIRIT MEDICINES

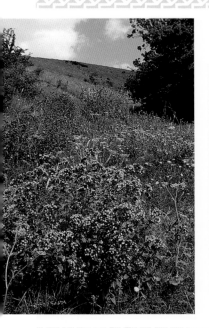

A versatile medicine, a tisane of marjoram relieves colds, coughs, sore throats, indigestion, and menstrual pain. It is an excellent remedy for fatigue with tension. Marjoram as a homeopathic remedy is

LEFT *Marjoram in flower – this useful herb grows in profusion and symbolizes warmth and happiness.*

indicated for nervous conditions and excessive sexual urges.

As a herb, it adds a sun-kissed flavor to vegetable dishes. Place a sprig in a bottle of olive or sunflower oil to create an aroma-therapeutic salad dressing.

As a flower essence, it brings support in times of danger and protection from harm. It calms, and releases fear. A few drops directly over your heart chakra will strengthen your faith in love and life.

Peony

LATIN NAME: *Paeonia officinalis*
FAMILY: *Paeoniaceae*

"My gift is to open your heart so you can express love."

From Greek antiquity to the Middle Ages, the peony was one of the most esteemed healing plants. With its many layers of flounced petals, the cup-shaped peony flower symbolizes honesty and truth.

SPIRIT AND SYMBOLISM

From tightly closed buds, peony flowers unfurl like hearts opening. The spirit of this feminine flower is sincere and loving. Native to China, where it is known as Sho-yu, meaning "most beautiful," the peony motif adorns temple walls for reasons told in an old Chinese tale. A scholar fell in love with a beautiful and talented woman. Sensing the approach of the eminent Chinese moralist, she fled, saying, "I am not a human creature, I am the soul of a peony, but your love warmed me into a human shape and now I must return to the human flowers." So her figure faded away, leaving only its image on the wall.

The peony was sacred to ancient Greeks, who regarded it as the first healing flower. Greek mythology tells how Asclepius, physician to the gods and also known as "paeon," or helper, received from his grandmother, Leto, a plant with which to cure Pluto after he had been wounded by Hercules. In Asclepius' honor, the plant was called peony and was a veritable cure-all.

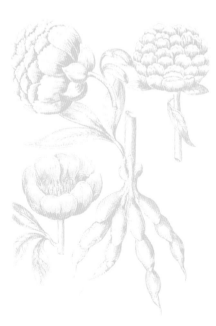

ABOVE *Flower of many parts – use the peony to soothe and reduce fever and pain.*

ORIGIN
The peony is a native of Greece and China.

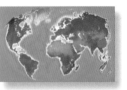

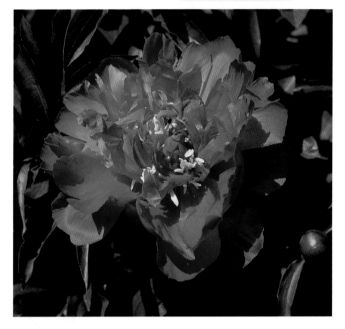

ABOVE *The beautiful sacred peony has been revered for its healing properties since the days of the Ancient Greeks.*

PLANT SPIRIT MEDICINES

In Chinese medicine, peony is cooling and anti-inflammatory. Decoctions of the root are used to treat fevers, swelling, pain from traumatic injury, night sweats, and muscle spasms.

As a flower essence, peony balances the heart chakra and encourages honesty in all forms of expression. It helps to dissolve away the false persona that many people have and brings the courage to present one's real self to the world.

American *and* Asiatic Ginseng

LATIN NAME: *Panax quinquefolius and P. ginseng*
FAMILY: *Araliaceae*

"I bring a gift of youth, endurance, vigor, and longevity."

For centuries this plant, or its man-shaped root, has been revered throughout Asia as an elixir of life. The masculine spirit of ginseng is the embodiment of strength, vigor, and virility.

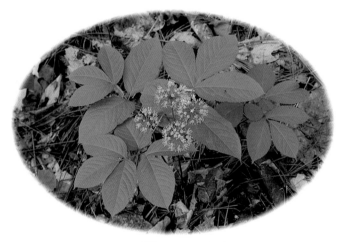

ABOVE *Life preserver – the ginseng plant may look nondescript, but it is highly valued for its properties.*

SPIRIT AND SYMBOLISM

This highly acclaimed panacea comes from a rather insignificant looking woodland plant that grows in the mountain forests stretching from Nepal to Manchuria. The name ginseng appears to derive from the Chinese, job-chen, meaning man-like. In the Far East, ginseng has always been the ultimate cure-all that prolongs life, bestows clear judgement, and enhances physical stamina. Chinese and Vietnamese troops are said to carry a root so that they are alert to danger and resistant to its consequences.

For countless generations the shamanic Laplanders of northern Scandinavia have relied on Nordic ginseng, known as kvanna, to help them cope with the extreme cold.

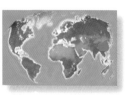

ORIGIN
The ginseng plant was found in both China and North America.

PLANT SPIRIT MEDICINES

In Chinese medicine ginseng is seen as harmony remedy that restores balance in a system overtaxed by stress and strain. As a herbal remedy, the roots are taken dried or their juice dissolved in alcohol to create a herbal elixir to prevent tiredness, exhaustion, forgetfulness, poor appetite, headaches, and the debilitating effects of old age.

Both kinds of ginseng bolster resistance to physical and mental stress, and contain substances that also act on hormonal systems. While Asiatic or Siberian ginseng is

BELOW *Dried roots of the ginseng are used to boost the tired body and encourage appetite.*

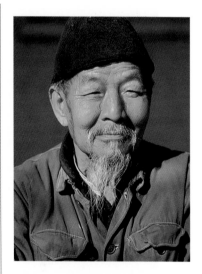

ABOVE *The ginseng plant has always been associated with longevity and improving the quality of life.*

good for body building and endurance sports, the American variety targets the nervous system, improves memory and learning, prevents circulatory problems and blood clotting, so reducing the risk of a stroke.

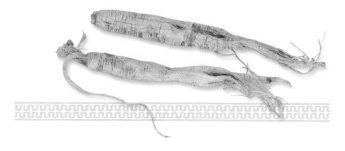

Opium Poppy

LATIN NAME: *Papaver somniferum*

FAMILY: *Papaveraceae*

"In healing heart pain, I calm the nerves and inspire dreams of wonder."

Historically, poppies have symbolized consolation in times of grief. With petals as fragile as tissue paper, the opium poppy also opens the doors to oblivion. Its spirit has a dreamlike quality that rekindles a sense of wonder.

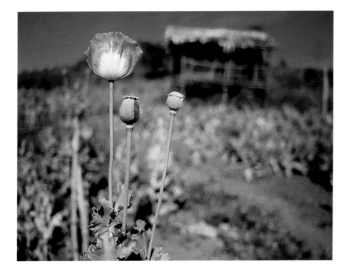

ABOVE *Somber but beautiful, the poppy symbolizes sleep and even death.*

SPIRIT AND SYMBOLISM

Originating from the Near East, the opium poppy yields one of the most powerful sleep-inducing narcotics known and since ancient times has been seen as a symbol of deep sleep, dreams, and even death. The ancient Egyptians used opium poppy juice as a dream-inducing narcotic.

In Greek mythology, when the gods see Demeter searching in vain for her abducted daughter they cause opium poppies to spring up around her. On swallowing their seeds, she falls into a deep sleep, putting an end to her anguish. Opium derives from the Greek *opion*, meaning poppy juice, while morphine gets its name from Morpheus, the god of dreams. All the nocturnal deities were crowned with poppy wreaths.

ORIGIN

The opium poppy is a native of the Near East.

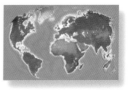

PLANT SPIRIT MEDICINES

The milky juice from the opium poppy provides the medical world with arguably its most valuable narcotics and painkillers – morphine and codeine. Tincture of opium, better known as laudanum, was once a popular sedative. So powerful are these preparations that they should never be taken unless under the strictest supervision.

White poppy as a homeopathic remedy is for shock with faintness, numbness, trembling, and eyes that appear glassy and stupefied.

As a flower essence, the spirit of the opium poppy helps to overcome addictions and deals with emotional states that lead to drug dependency. By rekindling our ability to dream and rediscover a sense of wonder, it alleviates the need to escape the real world.

BELOW *Powerful force – the poppy provides potent pain killers and sedatives.*

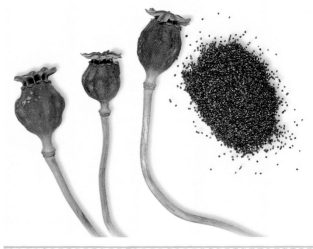

Passionflower

LATIN NAME: *Passiflora incarnata*

FAMILY: *Passifloraceae*

"I am the soul flower that holds the energy of divine consciousness. I help with the evolution of mankind."

An exotic climber with extraordinary flowers like works of art, passionflower grows wild in the damp forests of Central and South America. The flowers are best known for their tranquilizing properties, but their spirit inspires a more ethereal sense of the divine.

SPIRIT AND SYMBOLISM

Little is known of the native use of this plant, named in the seventeenth century by the Spanish conquistadors, who compared the emergence of this beautiful blossom from its unassuming bud with the Passion of Christ. In the intricate patterns of this flower they saw the five instruments of Christ's crucifixion – the hammer, spears, nails, crown of thorns, and pillar where He was lashed. Identifying the passionflower so closely with Christ, they assumed its presence was a clear sign that the natives would be ready converts to Christianity.

ORIGIN
The passionflower was first discovered in the South American forests.

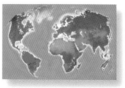

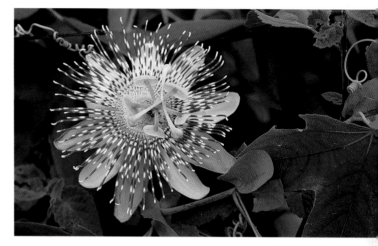

ABOVE *The outstanding beauty of the passion-flower has led to its symbolic place in Christianity.*

The spirit of this flower does mirror the divinity embodied by Jesus. Attuning to it evokes a sense of compassion, altruism, and unconditional love. In fact, the passionflower is frequently used as a religious symbol.

PLANT SPIRIT MEDICINES

As an infusion, passionflower tea is a gentle sedative for calming the nerves, relieving stress, and encouraging a good night's sleep. The fragrant flesh of *Passiflora edulis*, or passion fruit, has a pleasant sweetness that lends an exotic flavor when blended with other fresh fruit juices.

As a flower essence, passionflower stimulates pure, divine unconditional love. This in turn heals negativity, pain, and trauma. It frees physical tensions, bringing stability and eliminating emotional confusion so we can consider life's events calmly. Passionflower also opens the heart and throat chakras to higher or more spiritual levels of consciousness.

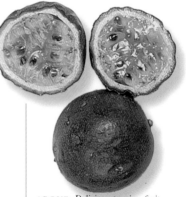

ABOVE *Delicious passion fruit, with its subtle flavor, makes a change from more common fruits.*

Date Palm

LATIN NAME: *Phoenix dactylifera*
FAMILY: *Palmae*

"I serve to remind you of the sweetness of life."

This lofty tree with its sprouts of feathery leaves is one of the most ancient food plants in the world. The date palm is deeply rooted in Middle Eastern culture and symbolizes an oasis of sweetness when life seems dry and barren.

SPIRIT AND SYMBOLISM

Equated with the tree of life throughout the Near and Middle East, the date palm has always been held in high esteem. The spirit of date palm is sweet-natured, tolerant of the harsher elements of life, and generous, bearing nourishing fruits in abundance. Sometimes depicted as the sacred tree on Chaldean cylinders dating back to 4,000 B.C.E., the date palm was undoubtedly worshipped

ORIGIN
*Dates originate from
the Middle East.*

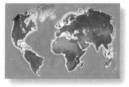

LEFT The Road to Jerusalem
by Fra Angelico (c1387–1455),
with date palms in background
and leaves on the ground.

as the embodiment of the supreme deity in ancient Assyria.

To ancient Egyptians, the date palm was sacred to the sun god Ra. They used the leaves for shelter, the fruits as a sweetener, and also turned the sugary liquid into liquors and wines. The leaves were most famously strewn in the path of Jesus when He rode into Jerusalem on a donkey.

LEFT *The date
palm has much to
offer, including
nourishment
and healing
properties.*

PLANT SPIRIT MEDICINES

Fresh or dried, dates are a nourishing food containing carotenes, B-complex vitamins, and an abundance of fructose, a sweet fruit sugar. They make excellent sweet snacks that are a wholesome alternative to biscuits, chocolate, and candies. In Islam, the fruits are **traditionally used for treating stomachache and heart conditions.**

As a flower essence, date is for bringing out feelings of tenderness, warm heartedness, and forgiveness. A good remedy for those who tend to be rather hypercritical, intolerant, and irritated by others.

PL. XXIV

FAMILLE DES PALMIERS.
le Dattier, *Phœnix Dactylifera.*

Frangipani *or* Temple Flower

ORIGIN
The South American tropics were the first home of the frangipani.

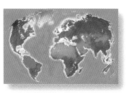

LATIN NAME: *Plumeria acuminata*

FAMILY: *Apocynaceae*

"I help to restore spiritual integrity and vitality."

In India, frangipani is seen as a most spiritual flower. Frangipani trees encircle small temples, filling the air all year round with a heavenly fragrance that evokes an atmosphere of serenity and profound peace.

SPIRIT AND SYMBOLISM

Frangipani, or temple flower as it is known in India, is a hardy tree with glorious white and yellow flowers with the most sublime scent that sends one's spirit soaring. Frangipani has been revered for at least 2,000 years by Polynesians, who believe it was created to enable the Pacific islanders to maintain and cherish the purity of their spiritual life and culture. On colonizing Hawaii, they brought their precious frangipani with them, and its blossoms are still threaded into the leis and garlands worn in traditional ceremonies.

In Indonesia, men and women partaking in ceremonies honoring the gods wear a frangipani flower behind their left ear to evoke an aura of peace and tranquillity. Women in India wear the flowers in their hair on all holy occasions.

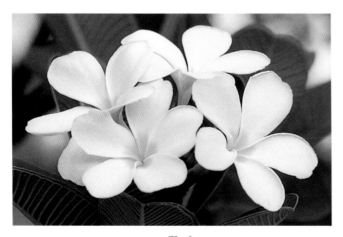

ABOVE *The fragrant frangipani is worn as a symbol of spirituality by Polynesians.*

PLANT SPIRIT MEDICINES

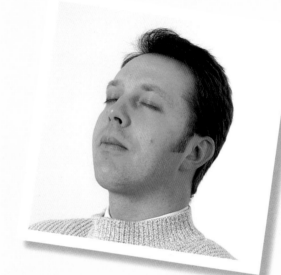

ABOVE *Relax as you inhale the intoxicating fragrance of the frangipani.*

To sense the spirit of this flower it helps to hold it and inhale deeply. The petals are smooth and waxy and its heady perfume can send you into a daydream far away from the hustle and bustle of life.

As a flower essence, frangipani helps to enhance, strengthen, and deepen spiritual worship and awareness of the divine. This is a remedy for those who have lost touch with their beliefs and feel alienated from their own inner spiritual values as a result of being caught up in another culture or a modern, materialistic society. On an energetic level it aligns the soul and causal bodies, integrating the wisdom of the soul with one's will-power.

Pasque Flower

LATIN NAME: *Pulsatilla patens*

FAMILY: *Ranunculaceae*

"I engender a feeling of protective love, release tension, and bring a childlike, carefree spirit."

With its pale lilac flowers, this small plant is a sacred power medicine of Native Americans. Flowering in early spring, the pasque flower embodies a spirit of youthful tenderness and joy.

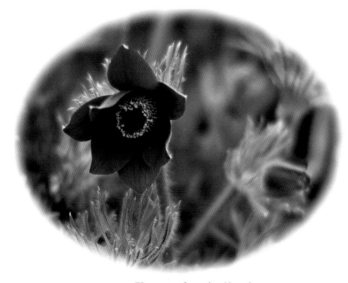

ABOVE *The pasque flower heralds spring and new life. Revitalizing and energizing, it is revered among Native Americans.*

SPIRIT AND SYMBOLISM

Known to the Omahas and Poncas as "little buffalo medicine," pasque flower is so precious that it may be used only by the medicine men of these two tribes. To them, pasque flower represents the spring of life and is associated with the south on the medicine wheel.

In Greek mythology, this flower sprung from drops of blood falling from the beautiful Greek god Adonis as he lay dying. Grief-stricken, Aphrodite beseeched Zeus to let him live again. He agreed on the condition that Adonis' time be divided between himself, Aphrodite on earth, and Persephone in the underworld. Adonis was celebrated as god of plants, his death and resurrection representing the regeneration of nature.

ORIGIN
The pasque flower is a native of North America.

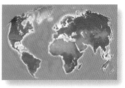

PLANT SPIRIT MEDICINES

A pasque flower tincture calms, soothes, and heals the nerves and provides a remedy for digestive problems, asthma, bronchitis, headaches, and nervous exhaustion. As a homeopathic remedy, *Pusatilla nigricans* (meadow anemone) is for symptoms of thick, yellow catarrh, swollen glands, and dry lips and mouth accompanied by emotional outbursts and weepiness. Most

BELOW *The pasque flower relieves many ailments, including headache and irritability.*

babies go through a *Pulsatilla* phase of being weepy, clingy, and whiny. Symptoms are always the better for fresh air.

As a flower essence, pulsatilla is for shy, timid, yielding, and overemotional people, who tend to be touchy and irritable.

BELOW *Associated with youth, the pasque flower helps maintain happy, healthy children.*

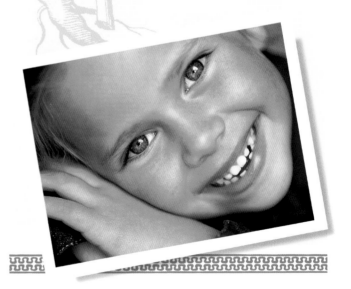

Pomegranate

LATIN NAME: *Punica granatum*
FAMILY: *Punicaceae*

*"I embody the essence of femininity and inspire
a celebration of womanhood."*

**Dressed in flaming shades of golden orange and
red, the flowers and fruits of the pomegranate have
long been a symbol of female fecundity. Break the
fruit open to reveal the sweet juices and seeds, a
reminder of woman's primary urge to create and
care for others.**

SPIRIT AND SYMBOLISM

The spirit of the pomegranate encapsulates the fiery and
creative aspects of femininity. Her gift is fertility. In ancient
Assyria and Babylonia, pomegranates were served at marriage
banquets to celebrate love and inspire fecundity.

In Greek mythology, Persephone was confined to the
underworld because she ate a pomegranate in the garden of
Hades. Her mother, Demeter, bargained with Hades, who
conceded that she could spend half the year with her mother.

ORIGIN
*The pomegranate originates from
Africa and the Near East.*

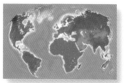

When Persephone is sepa-
rated from her mother the
countryside is sterile; her
return accompanies the
arrival of spring.

This symbolism
followed the pomegranate
into the Far East. At Asian
weddings, pomegranates
were thrown onto the floor
of the newlyweds'
bedchamber to bless the
marriage. Buddha said,
"Pomegranates will cleanse
your soul of hatred and
envy," alluding to their
warm and nurturing spirit.

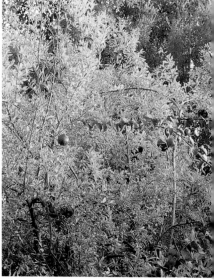

ABOVE *Symbol of fertility, the
pomegranate played an important part at
weddings in the Far East.*

PLANT SPIRIT MEDICINES

The pomegranate fruit
is a source of plant
hormones akin to
feminine hormones.
Eating fresh fruits
may smooth one's
passage through the
transitional, and
sometimes difficult,
phases of womanhood.
Stir their juice into
fruit punches and
sweet wines or
experiment with
grenadine, a
pomegranate syrup.
As a flower essence,
pomegranate
emphasizes all
the feminine qualities.
It kindles fire energy
and the primal urge to
create, procreate, and
care for others. This
essence also helps
women who feel
confused and
compromised as a
result of being torn
between career and
home life.

LEFT *The
pomegranate's
properties will
aid a woman
throughout her life.*

Oak

LATIN NAME: *Quercus spp.*
FAMILY: *Fagaceae*

"I work my magic by providing abundant resilience and inner strength."

Sturdy and sheltering, the majestic oak is the archetypal symbol of strength. The spirit of oak embodies the wisdom and fortitude that springs from having one's feet firmly on the ground.

SPIRIT AND SYMBOLISM

Oak is one of the most sacred trees and it was believed that oak was the first tree created by God. The Greek god Zeus was worshipped as an oak tree at Dodona, the oldest Greek sanctuary, where sacred knowledge and prophetic visions were sought. In the Iliad, Odysseus learns of "the plans of Zeus from the oak of lofty foliage." To partake of Zeus's acorns meant acquiring wisdom and knowledge.

ORIGIN
Oak was first found in both Europe and Central Asia.

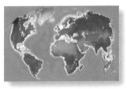

In folklore, the oak held the promise of fertility and prosperity. The Druids revered the oak above all others. The tree takes the human form of Sir Gawain, who as fertile summer does annual battle with the Green Knight of winter. In old England, maidens placed midsummer oak blooms under their pillows to dream of their future husbands, while acorns planted in darkness reputedly enhance fertility, bring prosperity, and protect from harm. In Greece, oak boughs were carried at marriage ceremonies and in West Africa women wishing for babies make offerings to their god, Loko, who dwells in the sacred iroko, or African oak (*Chlorophora excelsa*).

LEFT *Zeus, the king of the gods, was worshipped as an oak, which is "King of the Forest."*

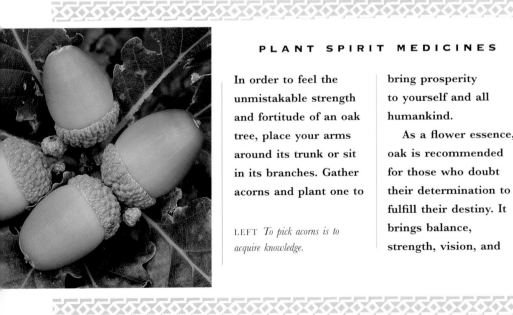

PLANT SPIRIT MEDICINES

In order to feel the unmistakable strength and fortitude of an oak tree, place your arms around its trunk or sit in its branches. Gather acorns and plant one to

LEFT *To pick acorns is to acquire knowledge.*

bring prosperity to yourself and all humankind.

As a flower essence, oak is recommended for those who doubt their determination to fulfill their destiny. It brings balance, strength, vision, and constructive action. Oak is also for reliable, responsible kind of people who shoulder their burdens without complaining, often taking on more than they can manage, which can lead to feelings of exhaustion.

Rose

LATIN NAME: *Rosa spp.*

FAMILY: *Rosaceae*

"With my blissful perfume I evoke the spirit of love from the heart."

With perfect buds that unfurl to reveal breath-taking beauty, rose symbolizes the essence of love. Her spirit is pure and divine, an inspiration for all that is true and enduring. She evokes an air of romance and the promise of pleasures to come.

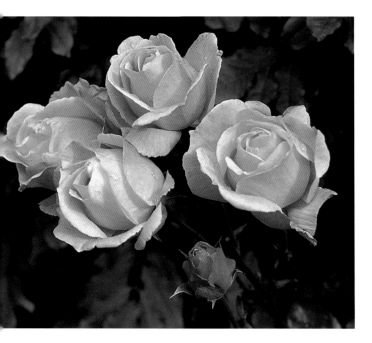

ABOVE *The perfumed rose has traditionally been associated with love and romance.*

THE SPIRIT OF THE ROSE

Her many petals portray a depth of personality and in the language of flowers different roses signify different characteristics or attributes. She is both inno-cent and seductive, delicate and strong. Her glorious, blushed flowers epitomize her femininity and youthful-ness. Few can resist the allure of a rose in full bloom; but be warned, her thorns will pierce those who treat her with disrespect. Native originally to the Orient, the rose in her many guises now graces gardens around the world.

ORIGIN
Roses were originally discovered in China.

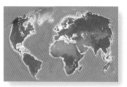

SYMBOLISM

In almost all cultures, the rose represents purity, perfection, and earthly and spiritual love. It is the flower of romance, seduction, and utter devotion. In legend, the rose adorned the earth thousands of years before the birth of mankind. Persians claim the rose was created from a drop of sweat falling from the brow of Mohammed. In Greek mythology, Dionysus fell in love with a beautiful nymph and as he pursued her through the garden, she tore her dress on a thorny bush, revealing more of her beauty. In gratitude, the god covered the bush in perfumed flowers, blushed rose-pink like the cheeks of his fleeing beloved.

From earthly infatuation and adoration of the divine, the rose symbolizes all forms of love. To the Sufis of mystic Islam, who transformed base metal of the soul into gold, the sacred rose symbolized divine love. To the ancient Greeks, the rose was sacred to Aphrodite, the goddess of love, worshipped in Rome as Venus. Today, the gift of a single red rose on St. Valentine's day still conveys a message of love and devotion.

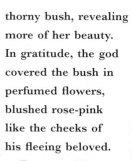

LEFT *The simplicity and beauty of an open rose is a powerful symbol.*

Rose

ESSENCE OF SPIRITUAL LOVE

The spirit of a rose is encapsulated in its flower extract. Envisage the rose flower fairy breathing her sparkling life force into this extract. By inspiring pure love, she helps us to rediscover the realms of the spirit.

• Gallica rose essence gives protection to fragile, oversensitive people and enhances the ability to communicate with the angelic realm.

• Centifolia rose extract calms and brings joy to the spirit.

• Green rose from China helps to develop, enhance, and spiritualize psychic abilities.

• *Rosa* x *alba* 'Alba Maxima' is a pure white rose associated with the earth or divine mother. It relieves problems arising from a lack of bonding with the mother and nurtures the child–mother relationship throughout pregnancy.

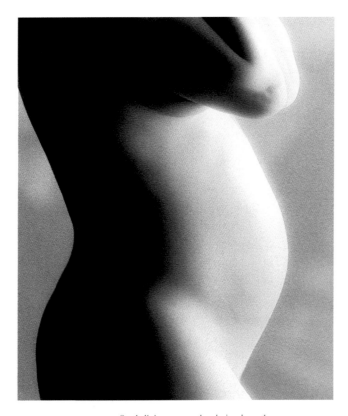

ABOVE *Symbolizing pure and enduring love, the white rose 'Alba Maxima' promotes the bonding process between mother and the unborn child.*

PLANT SPIRIT MEDICINES

Rose perfume enhances all that is feminine. It nourishes the heart, lifts the spirits, and evokes a sense of sexual bliss. As an essential oil (choose those distilled from *R.* x *centifolia* and *R.* x *damascena*), it is drawn to the female reproductive system, helping to relieve premenstrual tension, melt frigidity, and ease menopausal symptoms. Massaging the body with rose oil helps to stimulate circulation and preserve the youthful appearance of the skin.

An infusion of rose petals is good for the respiratory system and helps to treat coughs, hayfever, and sinus congestion.

RIGHT *Freshen your skin and mouth with rose water, made from rose petals.*

LEFT *Rose oil makes a perfect massage agent to encourage good circulation.*

Rosehips contain concentrated quantities of vitamin C and sipping rosehip syrup during wintertime affords protection from winter colds and flu. As a floral water, rose has mildly antiseptic properties and can be used as a refreshing complexion splash and a breath-freshening mouthwash.

Rosemary

LATIN NAME: *Rosmarinus officinalis*
FAMILY: *Labiatae*

"As an essence of remembrance, I help to evoke a memory of your own true path."

Rosmarinus, meaning "dew of the sea," thrives on sun-drenched slopes overlooking the vast blueness of the Mediterranean sea. Breathe deep her sweet aroma and remember inner truths that expand one's field of vision and reveal new horizons.

SPIRIT AND SYMBOLISM

An aromatic herb with shiny needle-like leaves and pale blue flowers, rosemary is for remembrance. Its spirit is loyal and constant, reminding us to stay true to those we love. Rosemary was once entwined in bridal bouquets and bridesmaids gave sprigs to the groom to symbolize love and loyalty. Greeks dedicated rosemary to Apollo, their solar deity, who was god of medicine, music, poetry, and prophecy.

Rosemary was burned as a purifying incense and carried in anti-plague posies to keep infection at bay. Gypsies hang

ORIGIN
The scent of the Mediterranean, rosemary also originates from there.

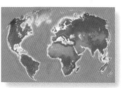

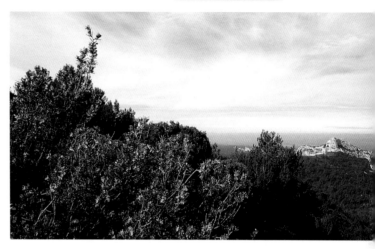

ABOVE *High above the sea in Provence, France, rosemary grows in profusion, spreading its delightful smell through the air.*

rosemary in their caravans to keep out evil and recommend putting a sprig under the pillow for protection and to prevent nightmares in children.

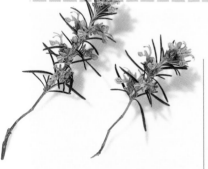

PLANT SPIRIT MEDICINES

LEFT *A most versatile plant, rosemary flavors food, relieves tiredness, and aids breathing.*

An infusion of rosemary flowers and leaves strengthens and revitalizes the whole system. It relieves weariness, promotes digestion, and soothes nervous heart complaints. In homeopathy, wild rosemary (*Ledum*) is for wandering pains and rheumatism.

As an essential oil, rosemary is strongly antiseptic and eases breathing problems, like sinusitis and asthma, when a few drops are sprinkled onto a pillow at night. Used as a room freshener, rosemary alleviates mental and physical fatigue. In beauty preparations, it promotes thick and lustrous hair growth.

As a flower essence, rosemary is for those who are forgetful, disoriented, and absent-minded because their spirit feels insecure. It develops clarity, sensitivity, warmth, vibrancy, and inner peace.

Willow *or* White Willow

LATIN NAME: *Salix spp. and S. alba*
FAMILY: *Salicaceae*

"I am a mystical guardian who bestows flexibility and optimism."

With her long weeping branches, the willow exudes an air of grace, dignity, and wisdom. Sit beneath her leafy canopy and feel her protective arms envelope you.

SPIRIT AND SYMBOLISM

Willow's whispering is often heard above the babble of a brook, for these trees have adorned river banks throughout Europe, Asia, and North America for centuries. Willows probably grew along the Euphrates, where they were regarded as the embodiment of Inana, the Sumerian goddess of life. To the Greeks

ORIGIN
The willow is a native of Europe.

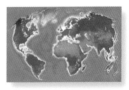

and Romans, willow was associated with Hecate, the fearless goddess of magic; with the moon and nocturnal journeys; with the moon goddess Selene (Luna), and also with Persephone (Proserpina), queen of the underworld.

Druids believed willow to be a magical guardian tree with a healing aura that blessed all she touched. The spirit of willow holds magical knowledge and in fairy folklore the spirit and elves living under willow's branches are keepers of herbal healing wisdom. In Native American tradition, red willow has special kinship with the spirit of the air. The Navajo Indians make wands, amulets, and prayer sticks from willow bark to use in sacred ceremonies.

LEFT *Moonrise over the Annapurna Mountains, Nepal. Traditionally willow has been associated with the moon and the night.*

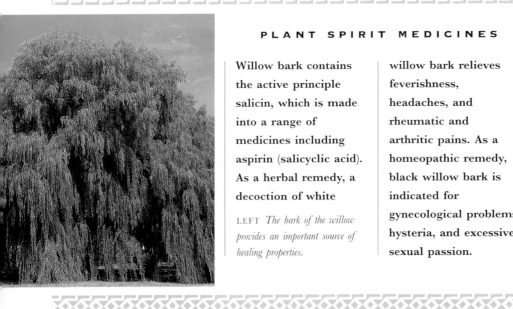

PLANT SPIRIT MEDICINES

Willow bark contains the active principle salicin, which is made into a range of medicines including aspirin (salicyclic acid). As a herbal remedy, a decoction of white

LEFT *The bark of the willow provides an important source of healing properties.*

willow bark relieves feverishness, headaches, and rheumatic and arthritic pains. As a homeopathic remedy, black willow bark is indicated for gynecological problems, hysteria, and excessive sexual passion.

The flower essence of willow inspires optimism and encourages a sunny disposition, while bringing mental resilience and receptivity. It is a good remedy for selfish, resentful, bitter people who bear grudges.

Sage

LATIN NAME: *Salvia officinalis*

FAMILY: *Labiatae*

"I help you to reflect objectively on the meaning of life and its spiritual dimensions."

With silken silvery leaves and pink or lilac flowers, sage is native to the sunny northern Mediterranean coast. Like its cousin mint, sage has the power to clarify the mind, which in turn helps us to see the greater picture that always exists.

SPIRIT AND SYMBOLISM

Salvia means to heal or save and the spirit of sage is like a guiding light that enables us to choose our direction wisely and find our way in the world. Esteemed since antiquity, the Greeks dedicated sage to Zeus and sipped sage tea to preserve memory and clarity of the senses, as they do today. Before China tea arrived in Europe, people enjoyed a daily cup of sage tea, while the Chinese, impressed by its power to relieve stomach problems, willingly traded 3 pounds/1.4kg of their tea for 1 pound/450g of sage. Druids believed eating sage leaves inspired wisdom, while folklore claims that the fairies and elves of sage charged the plant with energy that simply being near it subtly alters states of consciousness.

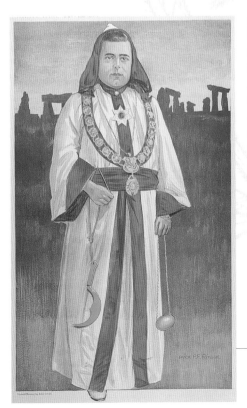

LEFT Chief Druid at Stonehenge Ceremony, *by Alick P. F. Ritchie in* Vanity Fair, *1911. Sage was an important plant to the Druids, inspiring wisdom.*

ORIGIN
Sage was first found in the Americas and southern Europe.

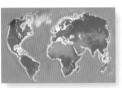

PLANT SPIRIT MEDICINES

As an infusion and tincture, sage is good for irregular menstrual cycles, frigidity, and menopausal symptoms. It relieves hot sweats, fluid retention, fatigue, and depression. Used as a hair rinse, a sage infusion imparts luster and shine. Chewing fresh sage leaves treats mouth infections, freshens breath, and cleans teeth, while sage tea makes a good gargle for sore throats and mouth ulcers.

Essential oil of clary sage (*Salvia sclarea*) added to massage oil helps relieve the same problems as sage

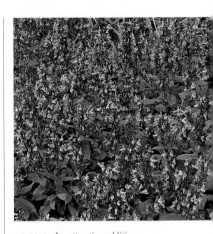

ABOVE *An attractive addition to a flower border, sage has many health benefits.*

infusion. A few drops in the bath helps treat liver congestion, thrush infections, cuts, and burns. As a homeopathic remedy, sage is indicated for night sweats and coughs. Sage flower essence helps us to comprehend the greater meaning of our lives.

LEFT *Fresh sage adds flavor to meat and freshens the mouth if chewed.*

Elder

LATIN NAME: *Sambucus nigra*
FAMILY: *Caprifoliaceae*

"I can help you to radiate the beauty and joy of youth."

Elder is one of the magical trees. Adorned with creamy white flowers that turn into sprays of dark purple berries, she has natural charm and elegance. Her spirit reflects the nature of true beauty.

ORIGIN
Elder is originally a European plant.

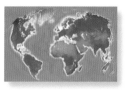

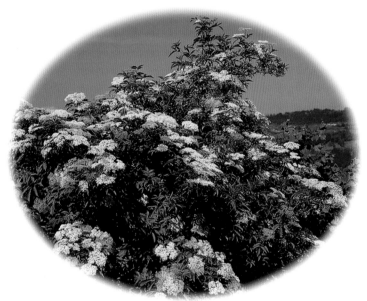

ABOVE *Elder flowers are infused for soothing colds. Berries make syrup to promote good health.*

PLANT SPIRIT MEDICINES

Remedies made from the flowers and berries make delicious spirit medicines. Flower infusions are soothing for colds, coughs, and hayfever symptoms. Use the stronger flower tincture to clear persistent congestion from the lungs and upper respiratory tract. A compress soaked in this lotion treats inflammation and infection in the eyes.

As well as easing sore throats and coughs, elderberries have been found to contain ingredients that stop viruses in their tracks. Sipping syrup of elderberries at the first sign of flu can nip the illness in the bud. As a flower essence, elder instills a sense of beauty and helps you to radiate the inner beauty that is within. During times of transformation and change, it preserves one's self-image.

BELOW *Pan pipes reputedly made from elder.*

SPIRIT AND SYMBOLISM

Throughout Europe and North America, elder has been seen as sacred. Folk legends refer to elders as places of refuge for good fairies and the home of a dryad "elder mother" who haunts anyone who chops down her wood. Remedies made from its flowers and berries were thought to bestow a long life, giving rise to the name "elder."

In Greek mythology, Pan, the sprightly god of fields, woods, and animals, plays pipes crafted from the branches of this youth-preserving tree. The druids used flower- and berry-laden bows in their wish-fulfillment rituals to bestow blessing and bring luck to young lovers. The elder is still hallowed by Gypsies, who will not destroy such a precious tree.

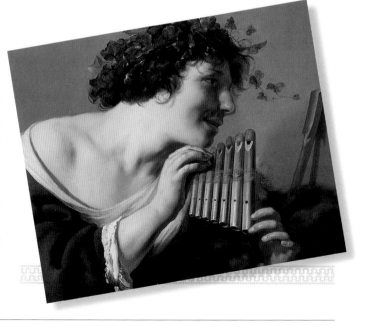

Sandalwood

LATIN NAME: *Santalum album*

FAMILY: *Santalaceae*

"I can flood your body with radiance and instil spiritual tranquillity."

On the hillsides of southern India where sandalwood grows, a divine perfume hangs in the warm air. Like a luxurious cashmere shawl, the scent and spirit of sandalwood wrap themselves around the very essence of one's being.

SPIRIT AND SYMBOLISM

The statuesque sandalwood with its leathery leaves and small purple flowers, emanates an air of peace and serenity. Like a child, it relies on other plants for nourishment in early life. In maturity, a strong sweet perfume pervades its dark brown wood, used to carve statues of deities and build temples. For centuries, Indian holy men have known that sandalwood clears and stills the mind, so the body and spirit can align as one. As an aid to prayer, meditation, and other spiritual practises, the scent of sandalwood fills Buddhist and Hindu temples throughout Asia.

Ancient Egyptians brought sandalwood from India and used the oil in embalming to help carry the soul of the dead into the next life, as well as in worship of their gods. Sandalwood has long been a main remedy of Ayurvedic medicine, the Indian system of healing that embraces the well-being of mind, body, and spirit.

ORIGIN
Sandalwood was discovered in India and southern Asia.

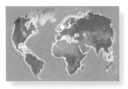

LEFT *With its pungent aroma invading the air, the sandalwood has been important in religious ceremonies in Asia and Ancient Egypt.*

PLANT SPIRIT MEDICINES

The perfume of sandalwood oil creates an air of sacredness and serenity that promotes meditation. As an essential oil, it soothes and relaxes, easing tension headaches, insomnia, nervous exhaustion, and depression. Sandalwood in massage oils calms inflamed and itchy skin conditions, such as psoriasis and eczema.

As a flower essence, the Hawaiian sandalwood heightens sensitivity to perfumes and deepens receptivity to aromatherapy oils. It energizes the crown chakra and enhances awareness of bliss.

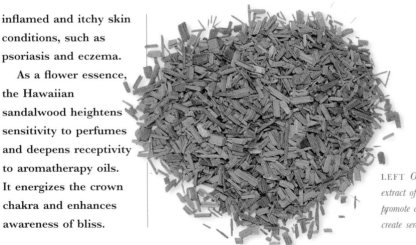

LEFT *Oil and extract of sandalwood promote calm and create serenity.*

Schisandra

LATIN NAME: *Schisandra chinensis*
FAMILY: *Schisandraceae*

"With my treasured berries I help the body and mind to adapt to stress."

Since ancient times schisandra has featured in Tibetan medicine as a superior herb with miraculous powers. This thorny bush with pale pink blossoms and ruddy berries has a spirit of youthful adaptability.

SPIRIT AND SYMBOLISM

Travellers to Tibet have been struck by the incredibly advanced age of many locals, who owe their youthful strength, energy, and alertness to schisandra. This plant is associated with Shangri-La, the legendary valley of everlasting youth which reputedly nestled in the Tibetan mountains. The magical secrets of schisandra have been known for nearly 5,000 years and it is described by Pen-Taso in the Emperor's ancient Yellow Book as one of the rare superior plants. Known in Tibet as "da-tring," schisandra is greatly revered as a youth-preserving tonic and fortifier.

ORIGIN
Schisandra is a native of China and Tibet.

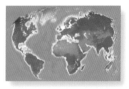

In northern China a hunting tribe called the Nanajs would carry dried schisandra berries with them before setting off on long trips in treacherous conditions. In the wilds of East Siberia, the berries, stalks, and roots are still drunk as a tea to provide extra energy to the hunters.

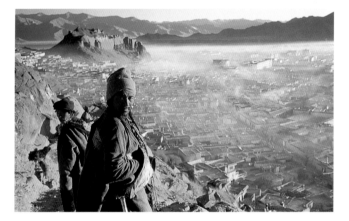

ABOVE *Shigatse, Tibet, the area associated with the schisandra herb linked to long life and energy.*

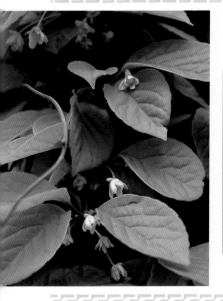

PLANT SPIRIT MEDICINES

LEFT *Schisandra promotes calm even at the most stressful times, maintaining the body's balance.*

Schisandra is one of the rare adaptogenic herbs that helps the body cope with all forms of stress. When taken as an infusion of berries, stalks, and roots, it maintains physical strength and stamina at times when one is pushed to the limits of endurance. Schisandra has a stabilizing influence on the nervous system and preserves a sense of inner strength and calm in times of anxiety. Schisandra's ability to help cells to utilize oxygen more efficiently means that it is useful to ease altitude sickness, reduce the need for sleep, and hinder the onset of exhaustion and fatigue.

Waratah

LATIN NAME: *Telopea speciosissima*
FAMILY: *Proteaceae*

"I give you courage to survive, no matter what."

Known by its aboriginal name, meaning beautiful, the magnificent waratah is one of the world's oldest flowers. To those who behold her beauty, she inspires bravery and a will to survive.

SPIRIT AND SYMBOLISM

An extraordinary looking plant with amazing red blooms comprising many tiny, tightly packed flowers, the waratah belongs to a genus whose origins date back 60 million years. Unique to Australia, the spirit of waratah embodies the bush-dwellers' qualities of adaptability and ability to cope in troubled times.

In Aboriginal folklore it symbolizes bravery and loyalty, as described in the tale of Krubi, a beautiful woman who lived with her tribe in the Burragorang valley. Krubi, who wore a unique cloak of red wallaby skins and cockatoo feathers, was deeply in love with a man who went off to fight for his tribe. Krubi sat alone on a sandstone cliff for seven days waiting for her lover, but he never returned and so she willed herself to die. As her spirit passed through a crack of sandstone a beautiful flower, colored in the same red of her cloak, grew in her place.

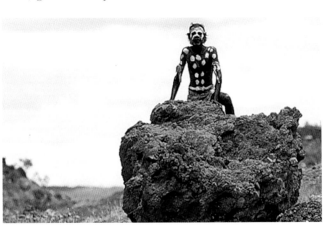

ABOVE *Used by the Aborigines, the waratah uplifts the spirit and aids recovery.*

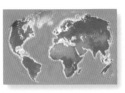

PLANT SPIRIT MEDICINES

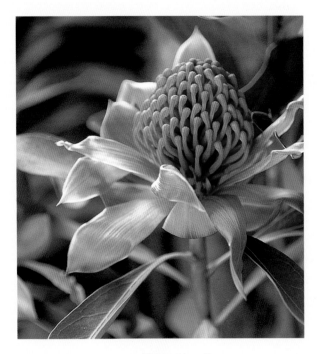

ABOVE *Native to Australia, the beautiful waratah is intrinsic to the Aborigine people.*

Waratah is traditionally used by Aborigines of the Tharawal tribe for its strengthening properties. The flowers are placed in a bowl of water so the nectar seeps out and the sweet liquid is used to treat illness in children and the elderly.

As a flower essence, waratah is a survival remedy. It brings courage, strength, and endurance to cope with change and major upheaval in life. A fast-acting remedy that dispels despair in those going through a time of darkness.

Thyme *and* Wild Thyme

LATIN NAME: *Thymus vulgaris and T. serpyllum*
FAMILY: *Labiatae*

"I enliven humor and bring joy to the spirit."

With its crisp aromatic scent, thyme exudes an air of lightness and brightness. Wild thyme can be found growing naturally throughout the Northern Hemisphere, from the sunny slopes of southern Europe to high in the mountains and in bitter Arctic regions. The spirit of thyme is lively and robust, embracing the harsher elements of life with joyfulness and enthusiasm.

SPIRIT AND SYMBOLISM

Garden thyme, *Thymus vulargis*, and its wilder cousin, *T. serpyllum*, are vigorous spreading shrubs that bear tiny pinkish-lilac flowers. Now cultivated worldwide, this refreshing herb has been used throughout history to brighten and purify the atmosphere. It was known to ancient Sumerians living 3,500 years ago and in classical times the Greeks used it to purify their temples and ritual spaces. To the Romans, thyme was sacred to the goddess Venus and was used in ritual baths to wash away sorrows of the past.

Druids scattered sprigs of thyme to bless the home and bring clarity and strength. Valued for enhancing psychic powers, it was used in spells for healing.

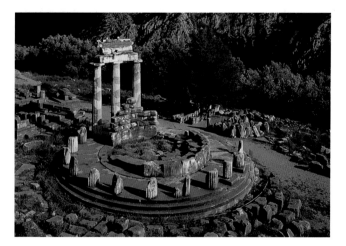

ORIGIN
Thyme has long been found growing in Europe.

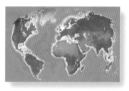

PLANT SPIRIT MEDICINES

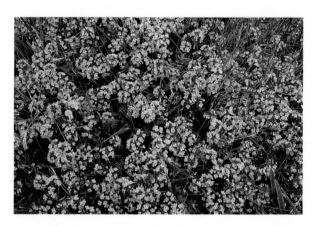

Thyme's therapeutic powers as a herbal remedy spring from thymol, a strong antiseptic. As a tisane or tincture, it helps to relieve bronchitis, hoarseness, chills, colds, nervous digestive problems, and tension headaches. As a compress, thyme treats abscesses, boils, and swelling.

As a homeopathic remedy, *T. serpyllum*

LEFT *The Temple of Athena, Delphi. Thyme was used in rituals in Greek temples.*

ABOVE *Thyme is a hardy and prolific grower, creating a carpet of light purple flowers.*

is recommended for children's chest complaints, nervous asthma, and whooping cough. Thyme flower essence lifts and brightens our spirits. It also alters our perception of time and is useful for past-life therapy.

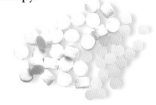

Red Clover

LATIN NAME: *Trifolium pratense*
FAMILY: *Leguminosae*

"With magic and luck, I bring health and wealth into people's lives."

It is said good fortune comes to anyone who finds a four-leafed clover. With its sweet, honey-scented flowers, the spirit of clover attracts all that is positive and rewarding in life.

SPIRIT AND SYMBOLISM

Clover is associated with luck and the phrase "living in clover" alludes to the good life symbolized by this cheerful plant. In folklore, the little green leprechauns of Irish mythology live in fields of clover, while the fairies that live in clover flowers are said to assist in finding love and kindness.

The Greeks likened the clover leaf to the triple-headed club carried by their hero, Hercules. To ancient herbalists clover was thought to be a god-given remedy.

Native to Europe and Asia, clover was first introduced from Britain into North America during the eighteenth century, where it was marketed by various Shaker communities as an excellent health remedy for aiding sound sleep and restoring fertility. Red clover was also made into a topical ointment for reducing lymphatic swelling.

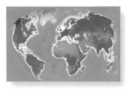

ORIGIN
Red clover is a native of Europe and Asia.

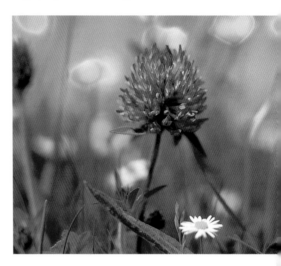

RIGHT
Representing good luck and cheerfulness, red clover is revered in folklore and mythology. It possesses special properties to speed recovery and promote good health.

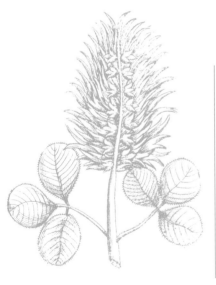

PLANT SPIRIT MEDICINES

LEFT *Whether eaten or cooked, or drunk as an infusion, red clover provides a range of health benefits.*

An infusion of the whole clover plant enhances the body's self-cleansing activity and speeds recovery from viral and bacterial infections. It is rich in plant hormones called phyto-estrogens that help to rebalance hormone levels and so provide some relief from menopausal and pre-menstrual symptoms. The plant also contains four compounds with anti-tumor activity and if consumed on a regular basis may afford some protection against cancer. Red clover can be steamed like spinach and used sparingly in vegetable dishes.

As a flower essence, red clover has magical qualities for stimulating inner strength and willpower and for clarifying one's direction in life.

Cat's Claw

LATIN NAME: *Uncaria tomentosa*
FAMILY: *Rubiaceae*

"I am the shaman-tree of the rainforest and my healing wisdom brings abundant health."

Cat's claw is a veritable treasure, unearthed from the Peruvian rainforests. The healing potential of this creeping vine, used as a medicine by the native Indians for several thousand years, is only just coming to light.

SPIRIT AND SYMBOLISM

The Ashinka Indian shamans, or medicine men, of Peru regard cat's claw as their most valuable medicinal herb for treating a wide variety of illnesses, including cancer. It has the strong, fighting spirit of a cat that refuses to give in to illness. Local Indians call it "uña de gato," or claw of the cat, because of its curved thorns. There are nine different varieties of this jungle vine; three look identical, but the local Indians

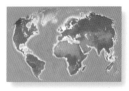

are able to identify, through subtle differences, the only species that possesses the healing powers.

The spirit of cat's claw is wise in the ways of healing and its red inner bark appears to work its miracles in various different ways. Native Indians call it "the Opener of the Way"

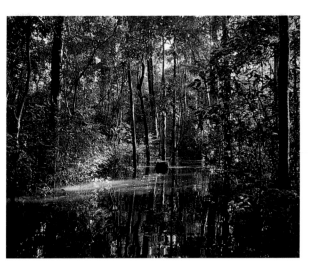

because cat's claw cleanses the entire intestinal tract. They see in this herb a power that helps those who are seriously ill to claw their way back to health.

LEFT *Cat's claw, creeping through the Peruvian rainforest, is an invaluable herb which has been in use for thousands of years.*

PLANT SPIRIT MEDICINES

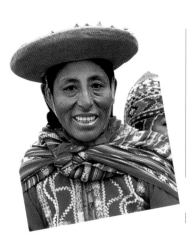

Cat's claw appears to have a beneficial effect on most health problems through its ability to stimulate the immune system and

LEFT *The most valuable of all the Peruvian Indians' herbs, the cat's claw aids immunity and is used to treat many illnesses.*

tone metabolic processes. A decoction of the inner bark is valued for its antiseptic, antiviral, and anti-inflammatory properties, making it a valuable treatment for chronic fatigue, depression, viral infections, gastric

upsets, arthritis, rheumatism, and even cancer. It may even exert a protective influence against heart disease. Native Peruvians wash wounds with cat's claw tea as well as drinking it to speed healing from within.

Vervain

LATIN NAME: *Verbena officinalis*
FAMILY: *Verbenaceae*

"Magically I purify mind, body, and soul, offering divine protection from all harm."

Once seen as a gift of God, vervain is one of the magical herbs. The spirit of vervain offers protection to those entering the world of enchantment and never lets us forget that dreams really can come true.

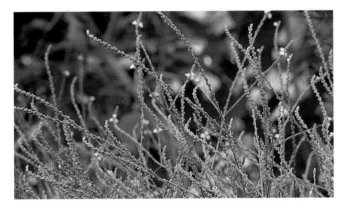

ABOVE *Revered throughout Europe, vervain has been used in religious ceremony and as a cure for fever and nervous disorders.*

SPIRIT AND SYMBOLISM

Worshipped by peasants in Greece and Italy, as well as the ancient Celts in Europe, this tall plant with pale lilac flowers derives its name from the Celtic word "fer," to drive away, and "faen" meaning stone and referring to heavy energies or toxins. Garlands and posies of vervain were worn as protection against witchcraft and mischievous fairy folk.

Vervain was considered sacred to Druids, the Celtic high priests. They cut vervain with a sacred sickle on the rising of Sirius, offering prayers of thanks and leaving a gift of honey to recompense the earth for her loss. They also wore crowns woven from vervain for protection when working with magic. Romans believed wearing or bathing in vervain afforded protection from Diana, goddess of the moon, and helped dreams come true, while priests and priestesses used small bundles of vervain to sweep and purify their altars.

ORIGIN
Vervain was found growing in Europe.

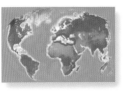

PLANT SPIRIT MEDICINES

A herbal tincture or infusion of vervain eases nervous disorders, asthma, and fevers. Applied externally, these preparations soothe inflamed eyes and as a gargle, they heal mouth ulcers and sore gums.

As a homeopathic remedy, verbena (blue vervain) is indicated for nerve-related conditions, such as insomnia, mental exhaustion, eczema, and psoriasis.

As a flower essence, vervain is a relaxing remedy for over-zealous, highly strung, or forceful people who try to impose their will and beliefs on others. This sets up stress patterns that vervain can undo.

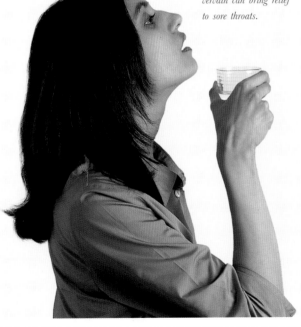

LEFT *Used as a gargle, vervain can bring relief to sore throats.*

Mistletoe

LATIN NAME: *Viscum album*

FAMILY: *Viscaceae*

"I can weave beautiful dreams of other worlds and unlock the mysteries of immortality."

Although mistletoe now invites a kiss at Christmas, in years past this unusual plant had protective powers and evoked dreams revealing the secrets of eternal youth. The spirit of mistletoe works in mysterious and magical ways.

SPIRIT AND SYMBOLISM

Mistletoe lives safely amongst the boughs of trees. With fine green leaves forming tiny horse-shoe shapes and almost irides-cent berries, mistletoe invites a sense of wonder.

This plant was sacred to Druids, especially when it grew in the venerated oak. Mistletoe cut with a golden knife at midsummer was used to strengthen magical work, provide protection, and bring healing.

In European folklore, mistletoe was hung over a baby's crib to stop mischievous fairies from taking the child. Placed above a bed, it inspires dreams of the secrets of immortality. In an old Italian tale, a beautiful fairy appears to a knight holding a sprig of mistletoe to which she attributes her eternal youth and beauty.

Mistletoe was brought into the home at Yuletide and a kiss exchanged beneath its leaves was thought to bring a blessing from the goddess of love.

ORIGIN

Mistletoe was found in Europe.

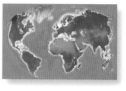

PLANT SPIRIT MEDICINES

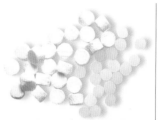

ABOVE *Mistletoe can help in the treatment of heart conditions and breathing difficulties.*

The berries are inedible, but mistletoe leaves contain active principles with promising anti-cancer properties. As a herbal remedy, mistletoe helps treat high blood pressure, but only when prescribed by a professional herbalist. As a homeopathic remedy, *Viscum album* is recommended for epileptic seizures, heart conditions, asthma, and complaints that are oriented to the left side of the body.

The flower essence of mistletoe helps to balance sexual energies with love. It also enhances the ability to maintain individuality within groups.

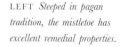

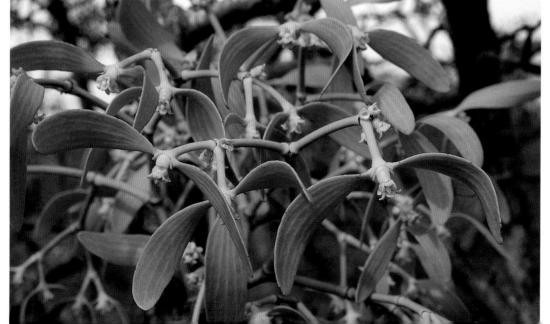

LEFT *Steeped in pagan tradition, the mistletoe has excellent remedial properties.*

Grape

LATIN NAME: *Vitis vinifera*
FAMILY: *Vitaceae*

"The joy of transcendence over human failings."

This vigorous vine with its distinctive leaves, curling tendrils, and succulent grapes, symbolizes the joy of living that comes from conquering our spiritual weaknesses as we pursue our individual path through life.

SPIRIT AND SYMBOLISM

The vine and its fruits represent a celebration of life. An old Persian legend tells how Prince Jemshed accidentally discovered wine when he drank fermented grape juice from his cellars. He drank freely, got a hangover, and thought the wine was poison. Feeling unloved, his neglected first wife sneaked to the cellar to poison herself. Instead the wine filled her with *joie-de-vivre* and the Prince fell madly in love with her again.

In antiquity, grapes and their wines were so important they were protected by deities such as Osiris in Egypt, Dionysus

ORIGIN
The grape originally came from Asia Minor and the Middle East.

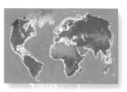

in Greece, and Bacchus in Rome. To the Israelites, grapes brought back from the Promised Land represented a new life, and in Islam, wine is the drink of the chosen in Paradise.

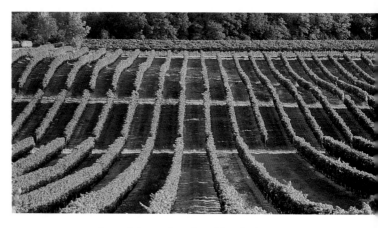

ABOVE *Rows of vines at Entre-Deux-Mers, Bordeaux, France, symbolizing a love of life and celebration.*

PLANT SPIRIT MEDICINES

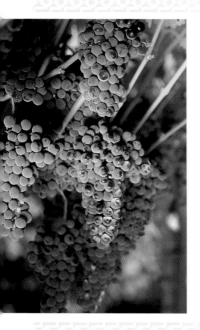

LEFT *Bursting with goodness, the grape cleanses, energizes, heals, and safeguards the heart.*

Grapes are rich in natural sugars and minerals, especially potassium and iron and are excellent cleansers. A one- or two-day grape fast can revitalize your whole system. Chemicals present in the leaves, grapes, and wine are potent antiviral agents.

In Chinese medicine, grapes are prescribed for blood and energy deficiency, as well as coughs, night sweats and rheumatism. A glass of wine brings relaxation, promotes digestion. Adding flowers and herbs to wine enhances its therapeutic action. As a flower essence, the spirit of the vine brings flexibility to those who are proud and dominating. It brings love without condition and patience with other's shortcomings.

Corn

LATIN NAME: *Zea mays*
FAMILY: *Gramineae*

"I encompass the nourishment of Mother Earth."

Wrapped in their lush leafy coverings, golden cobs of corn are a source of life-giving goodness and nourishment. To the ancients they symbolized wealth and plenty. As well as yielding a sweet and satisfying food, the maize plant has valuable medicinal qualities.

SPIRIT AND SYMBOLISM

Standing taller than a man, the maize plant delights in soaking up the sun. Its white and feathery flowers take both male and female forms, while its leaves are laden with cholorophyl, the green pigment that absorbs sun energy. In ancient times, corn was worshipped in male and female guises.

To the Mayan Indians he was the corn god, Cinteotl, and to the Hopi Indians Chalako-mana, the corn mist maiden. The Aztecs worshipped Veracruz as the corn symbol of fertility. In ancient Mexico, a corn plant is depicted with a humming bird symbolizing the Sun Hero and new growth.

ORIGIN
Corn is a native of the Americas.

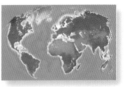

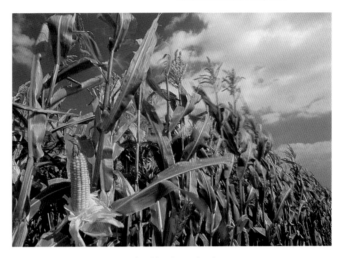

ABOVE *Sun-kissed corn has been revered across the globe.*

In ancient Greece, cornfields were tended by the goddess Demeter who represented peace, plenty, and fecundity. The Romans knew her as Ceres and the Druids as Ker, the corn mother who blesses and nourishes all her earth children.

PLANT SPIRIT MEDICINES

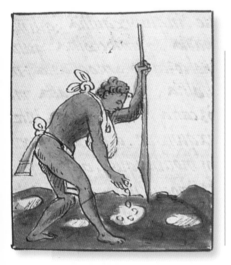

With its broad spectrum of nutrients, corn is a life-sustaining and body-building food. The leaves and inner silk have medicinal properties. Young

LEFT *From the* Florentine Codex, *mid 16th century, an Aztec man plants corn, to produce a valuable food and enhance remedial properties.*

tender leaves used as poultices are bound over wounds and sores to promote healing and draw out toxins. Used as a tisane, the silk treats kidney and bladder ailments, soothes prostrate gland problems, and prevents bed-wetting in children.

As a homeopathic remedy, cornsilk (*Stigmata maydis-zea*) relieves cystitis and kidney conditions. As a flower essence, corn rekindles mental, physical, and emotional energy for living life to the full by reconnecting us to the earth.

Ginger

LATIN NAME: *Zingiber officinale*
FAMILY: *Zingiberaceae*

"Like a catalyst, I ignite the vital fire, inspiring all into action."

Highly prized as a spice and medicine since ancient times, ginger pours its warmth and energy into every aspect of our life.

SPIRIT AND SYMBOLISM

With yellow flowers tinged with violet, the spirit of ginger is dynamic and fiery, qualities embodied in its roots that resemble tiny hands. Used in India and China for centuries for healing, ginger was one of the first spices to travel the silk route and was adopted by ancient Egyptians and Greeks who used it in cooking and to keep illness at bay.

To the natives of Dohu, a Pacific Island, ginger is sacred and imbued with magical healing powers. In an ancient ritual, the witchdoctor chews the root and then spits it onto his patient's wounds and burns.

In Hawaii, yellow ginger, or awapuhi, grows wild and bears exotically perfumed flowers that are woven into garlands and leis. As a lotion, awapuhi is traditionally rubbed on the head to relieve headaches.

ORIGIN
Ginger was originally found in India and Asia.

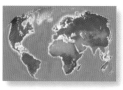

PLANT SPIRIT MEDICINES

Fresh or powdered ginger root used in cooking, fires the metabolism, stimulates the circulation, and aids digestion. As a tea, grated ginger sweetened with honey soothes coughs, sore throats, colds, chills, and nausea. In crystallized form, ginger may be sucked to relieve the nausea of morning and motion sickness.

Ginger essential oil diluted in vegetable oil makes a warming rub to ease swelling and rheumatic stiffness. The juice of yellow ginger is gargled to relieve a sore throat and applied to the scalp and hair as a beauty treatment.

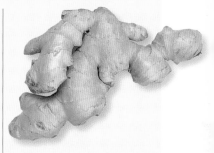

ABOVE *Ginger root spices up a variety of dishes and is beneficial to health.*

As a flower essence, yellow ginger encourages relaxation by releasing anger, irritation, frustration, and subconscious traumas. It is a remedy for enhancing sensitivity and perception.

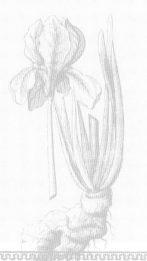

LEFT *Important in early trade, ginger has been used in cooking and as a remedy worldwide.*

RIGHT *As an oil or an extract, ginger soothes and heals.*

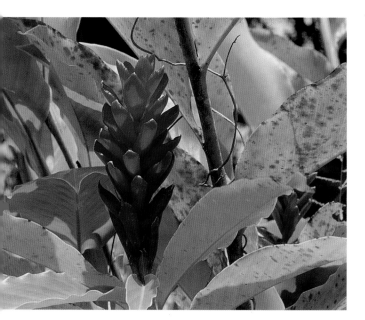

Bibliography

Adaptogens, Nature's Key to Well-Being, Mikael Wahlstrom, Skandinavisk Bok, 1997

Ancient Healing Secrets, Dian Dincin Buchman, Ottenheimer Pub., 1996

An Ancient Egyptian Herbal, Lise Manniche, British Museum Pub. Ltd., 1989

Aromatherapy in your Diet, Daniele Ryman, Piatkus, 1996

Aromatherapy – The Encyclopedia of Plants and Oils and how they help you, Daniele Ryman, Piatkus, 1991

Aromatherapy for Healing the Spirit, Gabriel Mojay, Gaia Books Ltd., 1996

The Atlas of Holy Places and Sacred Sites, Colin Watson, Dorling Kindersley, 1996

Australian Bush Flower Essences, Ian White, Findhorn Press, 1991

The Case of the Cottingley Fairies, Joe Cooper, Simon and Schuster, 1997

Chinese Herbal Medicine, Daniel P. Reid, Shambhala Publications, 1986

Chinese System and Food Cures, Prevention, and Remedies, Henry C. Lu, Sterling Publishing Co., 1986

Culpeper's Complete Herbal, W. Foulsham and Co. Ltd

The Druids' Herbal for the Sacred Earth Year, Ellen Evert Hopman, Destiny Books, 1995

Egyptian Mythology, Simon Goodenough, Tiger Books International, 1997

The Element Illustrated Encyclopedia of Mind, Body, Spirit, and Earth, Joanna Crosse, Element Children's Books, 1998

The Elixir and the Stone, Michael Baignet and Richard Leigh, Viking, 1997

Enchantment of the Faerie Realm, Ted Andrews, Llewellyn Publications, 1996

The Encyclopedia of Flower Remedies, Clare G. Harvey and Amanda Cochrane, Thorsons, 1995

Encyclopedia of Medicinal Foods, Joseph M. Kadans, Thorsons, 1979

The Fairies in Tradition and Literature, Katharine Briggs, Routledge and Kegan Paul, 1967

Fairy Spells, Claire Nabmab, Souvenir Press, 1997

Folklore and Odysseys of Food and Medicinal Plants, Ernst and Johanna Lehner, Tudor Publishing Co., 1962

Hawaiian Tropical Flower Essences, Penny Medeiros, My Island Publishing, 1995

The Healing Garden, Sue Minter, Headline, 1993

Healing Plants – A Modern Herbal, William A. R. Thomson, McGraw Hill Book Co. Ltd, 1978

Heaven's Mirror, Graham Hancock and Santha Faia, Michael Joseph, 1998

Herbal Handbook for Everyone, Juilette De Bairacli Levy, Faber, 1966

How to Meet and Work with Spirit Guides, Ted Andrews, Llewellyn Publications, 1997

The Illustrated Book of Signs and Symbols, Miranda Bruce-Mitford, Dorling Kindersley, 1996

Initiation, Elizabeth B. Jenkins, Piatkus, 1996

Larousse World Mythology, Pierre Grimal (ed.), Hamlyn, 1965

The Meaning of Flowers, Claire Powell, Jupiter Books, 1977

Medicine Dream, Marilyn Tunneshande, Hampton Roads, 1996

The New Oxford Book of Food Plants, J. G. Vaughan and C.A. Geissler, Oxford University Press, 1997

Neem. A Tree for Solving Global Problems, National Academy Press, 1992

New Vibrational Flower Essences of Britian and Ireland,
    Rose Titchner, Sue Monk, Rosemary Potter & Patricia Staines, Waterlily Books, 1997

100 Flowers and How They Got Their Names, Diana Wells, Past Times, Algonquin Books, 1997

Plants of Mystery and Magic, Michael Jordan, Blandford, 1997

Plants of Power, Alfred Savinelli, Alfred Savinelli, 1997

Principles of Vibrational Healing, Clare G. Harvey and Amanda Cochrane, Thorsons, 1998

Sacred Plant Medicine, Stephen Harrod Buhner, Robert Rinehart Publishers, 1996

The Sacred East, C. Scott Littleton (ed), Macmillian, 1996

The Sacred Tree, Mrs J. H. Philpot, Macmillan and Co. Ltd., 1897

The Secret Life of Nature, Peter Tompkins, Thorsons, 1997

The Secret Lore of Plants and Flowers, Eric Marple, Robert Hale Ltd., 1980

Shamanism, Nevill Drury, Element, 1996

Successful Herbal Remedies, Nalda Gosling, Thorsons, 1985

The Tree of Life, E. O. James, E. J. Brill, 19*6

West African Religion, a study of the beliefs and practices of the Akan, Ewe, Yoruba, Ibo, and kindred peoples,
    Geoffrey Parrinder, Epworth Press, 1969

Suppliers

U.K.

FLOWER ESSENCES
The International Flower Essence Repertoire
The Living Tree
Milland
Nr. Liphook
Hampshire GU30 7JS
Tel. 01428 741572/672
Fax. 01428 741679

NATIVE AMERICAN HERBS, COPAL, AND SMUDGING HERBS
Eagleheart
Middle Piccadilly
Holwell
Nr. Sherbourne
Dorset DT9 5LW
Tel. 01963 23468

CHINESE HERBS
The East West Herbs Ltd.
Langston Priory Mews
Kingham
Oxfordshire OX7 6UP
Tel. 01608 658862

MAJOR SUPPLIER OF MOST HERBS, ETC.
The Nutri Centre
7 Park Cresent
London
Tel. 0171 436 5122

SWEDEN

ADAPTOGENS
The Swedish Herbal Inst.
Viktoria Garden 15
S-413 14 Goteborg
Sweden
Tel. 31 77116778/7126136

FRANCE AND SWITZERLAND

FLOWER ESSENCES
Fleurs de Vie
The Flower Essence Company
Boite Postale 2
01170 Chevry
France
Tel. 450 42 62 32
Fax. 450 42 62 33
E-mail: orders@fleursdevie.com

Verlag Gesundheit & Entwicklung
Understadt 28
CH 8200
Schaffhausen
Switzerland
Tel. 52 624 63 50/624 50 30
Fax. 52 624 64 57

GERMANY

FLOWER ESSENCES
P.H.I. Korte
Hauptstr. 9
78267 Aach
Germany
Tel. 07774/7004
Fax. 07774/7009

U.S.A.

FLOWER ESSENCES
Flower Essence Pharmacy at Centergees
2007 NE 39th Avenue
Portland
OR 97212
Orders: tel. 800 343 8693
Tel. 508 281 4906
Fax. 503 284 7090

Flower Essence Society (FES)
PO Box 459
Nevada City
CA 95959
Tel. 530 265 9163
Fax. 530 265 6467

Aloha Flower Essences
PO Box 2319
Kealakekua
Hawai 96750
Tel./fax. 808 328 2529

CHINESE HERBS
East West Herbs Ltd.
6400 Hollis St.
Suite 10
Emeryville
CA 94608

SOUTH AMERICA

FLOWER ESSENCES
Essencias Flourais
Rua Alvaro
Rodrigues, 414 Casa 1
04582 – 001
San Paulo – SP
Brazil
Tel. 115317518
Fax. 112416063

AUSTRALIA

FLOWER ESSENCES
Rainbow and Bridges
68 Lynette Avenue
Warrandyte
Victoria 3113
Australia
Tel./fax. 398 44 2611

Australian Bush Flower Essences
45 Booratie Road
Terreyhills
NSW 2084 Australia
Tel. 9450 1388
Fax. 9450 2866

Living Essences of Australia
PO Box 355
Scarborough
WA 6016
Australia
Tel. 61 8944 35600
Fax. 61 8944 35610

Glossary

A

ACHILLES warrior-hero of Greek mythology, killed by an arrow which pierced his heel – the only part of his body not protected by a spell

ACUPUNCTURE the Chinese method of treatment in which needles are inserted in precisely chosen acpuncture points along the MERIDIANS to free blocked energy

ADAPTOGEN a substance that aids adaptation of the body

ADRENAL GLANDS two ENDOCRINE glands that produce adrenaline and various steroid hormones

ALCHEMY an early form of chemistry with the aim of discovering how to transmute base matter into gold and find the "elixir of life"

ALEXANDER THE GREAT king of Macedon, who founded a huge empire in the period 336–328 B.C.E.

ALKALOID nitrogenous compounds found in plants

ALTAI speakers of Altaic, a family of languages of Asia and South East Europe

AMINO ACIDS the substances that make up protein molecules, some of which have to be derived from the diet as they cannot be manufactured by the body

AMON Egyptian god of fertility

AMULET a bracelet or other piece of jewelry worn as a charm to protect from harmful spirits

AMUN alternative spelling of AMON

ANESTHETIC describes a substance that causes lack of sensation

ANIMISM the belief that all natural objects, large and small, animal, vegetable, and mineral, have their own spirits

ANTHROPOLOGIST someone who makes a formal academic study of human beings and their culture or cultures

ANTIBIOTIC a drug used in modern medicine to treat infection

ANTIFUNGAL having the power to destroy fungal infections

ANTI-INFLAMMATORY describes a substance or treatment that calms inflammation

ANTIOXIDANT a substance that prevents or slows down deterioration caused by the oxidation process

ANTISEPTIC having the power to destroy harmful micro-organisms

ANTIVIRAL having the power to destroy viruses

APHRODISIAC a substance that encourages erotic feelings

APOLLO the Greek god of healing (and also of music, light, poetry, and prophesy), associated with the sun

AQUEOUS CREAM basic, unperfumed preparation available from most pharmacists, which can be used in home-made skin creams

AROMATHERAPY therapeutic use of essential oils from plants

ARTEMIS the Greek goddess of the hunt and the moon

ARTHURIAN LEGEND body of legends of King Arthur of Camelot and his Knights of the Round Table (7th century)

ASTRAL BODY one of the subtle bodies surrounding the body

ATHARVA-VEDA an Indian sacred text

ATHEROSCLEROSIS a condition involving fatty deposits on the artery walls

ATTICA the territory of Athens in ancient times

AURA light, color emanating from living beings, usually visible only to those gifted in the perception of such things

AURIC FIELD the field of energy of the aura. This energy infuses the SUBTLE BODIES and reflects our inner vitality

AVALON island paradise in Celtic mythology (see CELTS)

AVESTAN one of the oldest Indo-European languages

AYAHUASCA a sacred visionary plant used in the Amazon

AYURVEDA an ancient system of healing from India, practiced increasingly today

AZTECS indigenous Mexican Indian people

B

BABYLON the chief city of ancient Mesopotamia

BABYLONIA kingdom of ancient Mesopotamia

BACCHUS the Roman god of wine, equivalent to DIONYSUS

BACH REMEDIES remedies based on flower and plant essences, discovered by the physician Dr. Edward Bach

BAEL or BEL Babylonian god also known as Marduk, the most prominent Sumerian god in the 13th–12th century B.C.E.

BALTHAZAR one of the three maji or wise men who brought gifts to the infant Jesus

BARASANA INDIANS a native people of Columbia

BEDOUINS nomadic Arab people of the Saharan Desert and other desert areas

BLOOD PRESSURE the pressure at which blood is pumped by the heart into the main arteries of the body

BO TREE the peepul tree or tree of wisdom, under which the Buddha gained enlightenment

BON the pre-Buddhist religion of Tibet (also the name of the priests of this religion), and now the Japanese Buddhist religion that celebrates the Feast of Lanterns

BORANA a people of Ethiopia

BRAHMA the Hindu creator god, one of the triad with Vishnu and Shiva

BUDDHA, THE the religious teacher Gautama Siddhartha (c. 563–483 B.C.E.), who founded Buddhism

BUDDH GAYA Indian sacred site and pilgrimage center where the Buddha received enlightenment

BUDDHISM the religion stemming from the East that has as its end the attainment of enlightenment by overcoming greed, hatred, and delusion

C

CALCIUM an element needed for the development and maintenance of healthy bones and teeth, and for healthy blood clotting

CAROTENE the orange pigment in fruits, vegetables, and egg yolk that enables the body to make vitamin A

CAUSAL BODY one of the SUBTLE BODIES surrounding the body

CELESTIAL BODY one of the SUBTLE BODIES surrounding the body, also called soul body

CELTS Indo-European people who inhabited Britain and parts of west and central Europe in pre-Roman times

CEREMONY respectful performance of a ritual

CHAKRA energy vortices situated at the center of the body that transform, transmit, and receive energy. There are seven chakras, inextricably linked to the meridian system in Chinese medicine: root or base, hara, solar plexus, heart, throat, third eye, and crown chakras

CHALDEA or CHALDAEA an alternative name for BABYLIONIA in the period c. 6th–5th century B.C.E.

CHARAKA an Indian herbal or pharmacopeia

CH'I the energy flowing through all living things in the thinking of Chinese philosophy and medicine

CHILU the notion of LIFE FORCE in the BON religion

CHULA the notion of LIFE FORCE in the ALTAI tradition

CLEOPATRA queen of Egypt from c. 70–30 B.C.E.

COPAL RESIN the RESIN obtained from various tropical trees

COMPRESS a pad soaked in a plant INFUSION or DECOCTION to be pressed against a sore or injured part of the body

CULPEPER, NICHOLAS author of *The English Physician Enlarged* (1653), one of the best-known English herbals

D

DECOCTION a plant extract made by simmering the plant parts (usually seeds, roots, or bark) briefly in water

DESPACHO CEREMONY ceremony of the Q'UEROS in honor of Pachamama, the earth mother

DEVAS gods or divine beings in Hindu and Bhuddist world-views

DIGITALIS a modern heart drug prepared from dried leaves and seeds of foxglove plants

DIONYSUS the Greek god of wine

DIOSCORIDES a Greek physician of the 1st century who worked in Rome. His *Materia Medica* (listing therapeutic drugs) was a standard work until the early 17th century.

DIURETIC a substance that encourages the flow of urine

DOCTRINE OF SIGNATURES a doctrine of medieval herbalists to the effect that the appearance of a plant provides the clues to its healing powers

DOGON a people of West Africa

DREAMTIME a sacred time-realm in Aborigine belief, which is entered through chanting and dancing ceremonies

DRUID a priest-magician in ancient Britain, Gaul, and Ireland

DRYAD a woodland spirit in Greek mythology (the word comes from the Greek *drus*=tree)

E

EA Sumerian god of water and wisdom

EDEMA swelling caused by excess fluid in the tissues

ELIXIR liquid medicine containing a sweet syrup to mask the taste; also a "sovereign" or outstanding remedy, as produced by alchemy; a remedy that gives long or everlasting life

ELYSIUM the dwelling place of the blessed after death in Greek mythology, also called the Elysian Fields

EM HAIN ethereal dwelling place of the blessed

EMOTIONAL BODY one of the subtle bodies surrounding the body

ENDOCRINE SYSTEM the complex system whereby the various endocrine glands release hormones into the bloodstream

ENERGY SYSTEMS all the subtle systems – the aura, chakras, subtle bodies, and meridians – that contain and transport energy

ENZYMES groups of proteins that act as catalysts in biochemical reactions such as those involved in digestion

ESSENTIAL OILS fine, perfumed oils that can be extracted from flowers and other parts of plants

ETHEREAL ENERGY invisible but perceptible spirit energy

ETHERIC BODY the layer of energy or SUBTLE BODY surrounding the body, lying closest to the body

ETHERIC ENVELOPE the outer layer of the SUBTLE BODIES surrounding the body

ETHNOBOTANISTS botanists who study the use of plants in folklore and religion, especially in other cultural traditions

EUPHRATES one of the two rivers flowing into the Persian Gulf, whose fertile valleys allowed early forms of civilization to flourish

EXFOLIATOR a treatment or substance that removes the outer layer (e.g. of skin)

EXTRAORDINARY MERIDIANS extra energy channels in the Chinese MERIDIAN system, linked to the main meridians, chakras, and subtle bodies.

F

FAERY old spelling of fairy

FLOWER ESSENCE the healing energy of a flower, transmitted to dew that has settled on the blossom or to pure water in which it has been steeped. This essence is used as a remedy

G

GAIA the earth goddess in Greek mythology

GAUTAMA see BUDDHA, THE

GAWAIN one of the Knights in the ARTHURIAN LEGENDS

GITCHI MANITOU the Great Spirit of Native North American myth

GLYCOSIDES substances derived from plants and used to make pharmaceutical drugs

H

HADES another name for PLUTO

HALLUCINOGENIC describes a substance that causes hallucinations

HAMMURABI the King of Babylonia in c. 18th century B.C.E.

HATHOR Egyptian earth goddess

HEALING CRISIS a stage often experienced in natural healing, during which symptoms temporally worsen (see also TOXIC RELEASE)

HEMORRHAGE bleeding, which may be internal or external

HENBANE the poisonous plant *Hyoscyamus niger* associated with witchcraft

HERACLES a Greek hero, performer of twelve impossible-seeming labors; also known as Hercules

HERODOTUS Greek historian (c. 485–425 B.C.E.), known as the Father of History

HESPERIDES the islands of the Blessed in Greek mythology

HINDUISM the dominant religion of India, in which the Brahma is worshiped as the supreme being and which includes belief in reincarnation and the worship of many gods

HIPPOCRATES the Greek physician, practising c. 400 B.C.E., known as the Father of Medicine

HOMEOPATHIC DILUTION a remedy prepared by repeatedly diluting the original substance in a carefully regulated way

HOMEOPATHY system of medicine, which works on the principle that patients can be cured by infinitessimal doses of a substance that would normally cause symptoms of their disease

HOMER ancient Greek poet living c. 800 B.C.E.

HORMONE-BALANCING describes powers in a plant or plant medicine to restore normal hormone balance

HORUS falcon god of ancient Egypt, later identified as the sun god

I

I CHING Chinese book of wisdom and divination

ILIAD epic Greek poem attributed to HOMER describing the Trojan wars

IMMUNE SYSTEM the complex system whereby the body protects itself from infection by invading microorganisms

INCA the South American indigenous culture of Peru that lasted from c. 1100 C.E. until the Spanish conquest of the 16th century; also the rulers of the Inca empire

INFUSION a tea made by steeping plant parts in very hot water for a short time

IROKO an African hardwood tree,

also known as loko

ISHTAR the principal goddess of ancient Babylon and Assyria, deity of love, fertility, and war

ISIS Egyptian fertility goddess

J

JINNI (plural JINN) a spirit capable of assuming human and animal form and able to influence people (Muslim mythology)

JOSEPHUS Joseph ben Matthia, a Jewish historian who lived c. 37–100 C.E.

K

KANE the god of creation in Hawaiian mythology

KI the Japanese term for QI or CH'I

KIKUYU a people of East Africa

KURAK South American priest or shaman from the Q'ueros tribe

L

LANCELOT one of the Knights of King Arthur in ARTHURIAN LEGEND

LIFE ESSENCE the distinct energy of any living being, whether animal or plant

LIMBIC SYSTEM the "primitive" part of the brain centring on emotions, hunger, and sex, and very responsive to scent

LINOLEIC ACID an essential fatty acid

LYMPHATIC SYSTEM the network of vessels carrying lymph fluid (involved in fighting disease) round the body

M

MANA is the spiritual life force in Hawaiian mythology, a creative aspect of the god Kane

MANTAS ceremonial tools used by the Kurak in Q'ueros tribal rituals

MASAI warrior tribe of Kenya and Tanzania

MATAGORA plant viewed as an elixir of life in the ALTAI tradition

MAYA the Native American culture whose golden age was from c. 300–600 C.E. and which flourished until the Spanish conquest

MEDICINE WHEEL a sacred ceremony of Native North Americans, symbolizing the circle of life, performed to aid in obtaining spiritual knowledge

MEDITATION a contemplative process which releases us from our everyday thoughts, leading to altered states of consciousness and enhanced powers of perception

MENTAL BODY one of the subtle bodies surrounding the body

MERIDIANS channels of energy in the body, each associated with a different organ, in the ancient system of Chinese medicine

MESCALINE a hallucinogenic drug obtained from mescal, the peyote cactus

MESITZO a native people of Peru

MESOPOTAMIA a region in the area of the Tigris and Euphrates rivers, sometimes known as the "cradle of civilization" because of its ancient cultures

MESOZOIC relating to the era from 225–155 million years ago

METABOLIC PROCESS the processes whereby food is used by the body

MIKO a female shaman of the SHINTO religion

MINOANS Bronze Age inhabitants of Crete, c. 3000–1100 B.C.E.

MOSES Old Testament prophet and Hebrew leader

MOTHER TINCTURE see TINCTURE

N

NANGSHEN purification rituals in the BON religion

NARCOTIC any consciousness-dulling substance

NATUROPATHY nature cure treatments

NEANDERTHALS early people living in the Paleolithic, the period up till about 12,000 B.C.E. during which primitive man emerged

NEFERTITI Egyptian queen of the 14th century B.C.E.

NEOLITHIC the New Stone Age, the period beginning in south-west Asia c. 9000–6000 B.C.E.

NEUROLOGICAL SYSTEM another term for the network of nerve cells that forms the nervous system

NICOTINE the alkaloid found in tobacco

NUT Egyptian sky goddess

NYMPH a nature spirit in the form of a beautiful young girl

NYOONGAH native people of South West Australia

O

OHARAI ritual ceremony of purification in the SHINTO religion

OPIATE a substance that induces dulled senses or trancelike state; a NARCOTIC

OSHA a plant used by the Sioux, known as bear medicine

OSIRIS Egyptian god of the underworld

P

PACHAMAMA sacred earth mother in South American cultures

PANYA physical reality in the tradition of the Q'ueros

PAPYRUS an Egyptian scroll or document (plural PAPYRI)

PARACELSUS a controversial and innovatory Austrian medical practitioner and theoretician (1493–1591)

PARASYMPATHETIC NERVOUS SYSTEM the part of the nervous system responsible for unconscious control of bodily function, such as rate of heart beat

PARATHYROID any of several hormone-secreting glands within the thyroid. The parathyroid hormone they release controls the level of blood calcium

PEEPUL another name for the holy bo tree

PERICARDIUM one of the "organs" referred to in Chinese medicine (not corresponding to a bodily organ as recognized in Western medicine)

PERICLES Athenian statesman who died in 429 B.C.E.

pH a measure of acidity or alkalinity

PHARMACIST someone trained to prepare and dispense drugs and medicines

PHARMACOPEIA official list of medicinal drugs or plants and their uses

PHYTO-HORMONES hormones or hormonelike substances, such as estrogen and progesterone, found in plants

PHYTOTHERAPIST a therapist who uses plant medicine

PINEAL GLAND the gland, situated in the brain, thought to be involved in the secretion of melatonin

PIPAL alternative spelling for PEEPUL

PITUITARY GLAND the chief of the ENDOCRINE GLANDS, situated in the brain, and controlling the functioning of the other endocrine glands

PLANT SPIRIT MEDICINE remedy inspired by the spirits of healing plants

PLINY THE ELDER the Roman author of *Natural History,* who lived 23–79 B.C.E.

PLUTO the Greek god of the underworld

POTASSIUM SALTS source of potassium in the body, an important element, which has to be balanced by sodium

POULTICE a form of COMPRESS of fresh or dried herbs made into a paste

POPUL VUH a sacred text of pre-Hispanic Mexico

PRANA the vital energy or life force in Ayurvedic medicine (see AYURVEDA)

PSORIASIS a skin condition in which the cells of the epidermis reproduce too quickly, causing itching, scaling, and red blotches

PSYCHEDELIC mind-altering or perception-changing

PSYCHOSOMATIC describes states of the body that are linked to mental states or emotions

PTAH Egyptian god, thought of as the creative power

PULSE RATE the rate at which blood flows in the blood vessels, and also the vibrations of forms of energy flowing through the chakras and meridians

PYTHAGOREANS followers of Pythagoras, the Greek mystic, philospher, and mathematician who lived c. 580–500 B.C.E. They studied the mathematical relationships inherent in the universe and lived an ascetic and religious life

Q

QI alternative spelling of CH'I

QI GONG a Chinese system of contemplative exercise by which energy is balanced and enhanced

Q'UEROS an indigenous people of Peru

QUETZALCOATL Aztec and Toltec god in the form of a feathered serpent

QUININE an extract from chinchona bark, used to treat malaria and fevers

R

RA the Egyptian sun god

RAINBOW SNAKE the creator spirit of the NYOONGAH people

RAMSES III king of Egypt who died c. 1167 B.C.E.

RESIN a gummy substance exuded from trees and other plants

RIG-VEDA a sacred Indian text

S

SACRED BUNDLE selected flowers, herbs, or other plant pieces formed into a bundle and carried to protect and heal

SACRED SMOKE ceremonial burning of sacred plants

SAKAKI sacred tree in the SHINTO religion

SALICIN an analgesic substance obtained from willow and poplar tree bark, from which aspirin is developed

SANSKRIT the ancient language of India, as used in the Vedic scripts

SHAMAN a healer-priest or medicine man – or woman

SHAMANISM religion of northern Asia and Native North Americans, in which a priest or medicine man (the shaman) can influence spirits for the benefit of human beings' health and good fortune

SHINTO the indigenous religion of Japan

SHIVA Hindu destroyer god, one of a triad with Brahma and Vishnu

SINUSITIS an inflamed condition of the mucous membranes lining the sinuses, as in hayfever

SIOUX an indigenous native people of North America

SIRIUS the dog star

SMUDGE STICK a bundle of herbs or plant pieces used in the Native North

American SMUDGING CEREMONY

SMUDGING CEREMONY the ceremonial burning of sacred plants to cleanse a physical and mental space

SOCOTRA an Indian Ocean island

SOLOMON king of Israel in the 10th century B.C.E.

SOMA an intoxicating drink made of plant juice and used in Vedic rituals

SPIRIT ENERGY the subtle forms of energy that give plants their healing powers

SPIRITUAL BODY one of the SUBTLE BODIES surrounding the body, also called illuminated body

SPIRITUAL ESSENCE the essence of our non-physical being, which emanates from the combined energies of the SUBTLE BODIES

STEAM INHALATION method of treatment in which the patient inhales vapors from an INFUSION

STEROIDS organic compounds, many of which have significant physiological effects

SUBTLE BODIES the layers of energy surrounding the body, divided into etheric, emotional, mental, and astral bodies

SUFIS members of a mystical Muslim sect

SUMER the site (in MESOPOTAMIA) of the world's first civilization c. 3400 B.C.E.

SUNDANCE CEREMONY an initiation ceremony of Native North Americans

SUTRAS Sanskrit writings on Vedic doctrine

SWEAT LODGE CEREMONY a Native North American healing ceremony, performed to purify the spirit

SYLPH a woodland spirit in the form of a young girl

T

TABOO something that is forbidden by ritual (and usually held sacred)

T'AI CHI a Chinese system of flowing movements that balance energy, linked originally to martial arts

TAOISM the philosophy of the ancient Chinese teacher Lao-tse, which developed into a popular religion incorporating the idea of nature spirits and sorcery

TEEPE an animal-skin tent used by Native North Americans to live in

THERAPEUTIC a substance or form of treatment with the power to cure

THROMBOSIS the clotting of the blood within an artery or a vein

THYMUS a gland just below the thyroid, involved in the development of immune responses in childhood

THYROID a gland that secretes hormones involved in metabolism and growth control

TINCTURE a preparation made by steeping the plant material (or other materials used) in alcohol. A few drops are then mixed with water for use. Flower essences can be preserved in this form (often known as the "mother tincture")

TINNITUS a condition whose symptoms are roaring or hissing noises in the ears

TIR NA OG mythical realm of the fairies

TISANE an infusion or herbal tea

TOXIC RELEASE the often unpleasant early stages of healing when the body is releasing toxins

TRIPLE WARMER one of the "organs" of the body in Chinese medicine, with no counterpart in Western medicine

TUTANKHAMUN Egyptian Pharaoh ruling c.1352–1342 B.C.E., who restored the worship of AMON

U

UNICORN a mythical one-horned horse-like animal

V

VEDA the sacred writings of Hinduism

VEDIC adjective from VEDA

VERTIGO dizziness

VESICLE a blister-like sac or cavity containing a liquid

VIBRATIONAL responsive powers of flowers and plants and plant medicine, not yet scientifically explained, relating to energy within plants

VISHNU Hindu god, the Sustainer, one of a triad with Brahma and Shiva

VISUALIZATION a technique of purposeful, controlled day-dreaming

VITAL FORCE the life energy in theories of homeopathy, similar to the idea of CH'I in Chinese medicine

W

WAQ the supreme god of the BORANA people

WITCHDOCTOR shaman or medicine man, especially in Africa

Y

YANG one of the two complementary and opposing forces operating throughout the universe at every level, according to theories of Chinese philosphy and medicine; the counterpart of YIN

YIN the counterpart of YANG

YOGI an Indian wise man, literally a master of yoga

YOQE invisible reality in the traditions of the Q'UEROS

Index

Acknowledgments from Clare Harvey

To Burgs for his love and enthusiasm.

To Susan Mears (my agent) for her care and support.

A heartfelt thanks to Peruvian Shaman Mateo and Andean Shaman Cucho
for sharing their insight, wisdom, and for opening the door to the plant spirit world.

To Hyemeyohsts and Swan Storm (Mayan Tradition),
Merilyn Tunneshende (Nagual Tradition), and
Jamie Sams (Native American Tradition)
for their wonderful teaching.

To Jerry Wills (Great Expeditions)
for sharing his jungle and vision with me.

To Penny Medeiros (Aloha Hawaiian Flower Essences),
Ian White (Australian Bush Essences),
Andreas Korte (Amazonian Orchid Essences),
Eliana Harvey (White Eagle Medicine Cards),
Colette Prideaux-Brune (Aromatherapy), and
Deborah Vear (Herbalism)
for their invaluable advice and friendship.

A special thanks to the tiny wondrous spirit-beings that aided and inspired this project.

Acknowledgments from Amanda Cochrane

My thanks go to Sue Cochrane for providing valuable insights into African beliefs and healing traditions
and for supplying a wealth of original reference material.

To Daniele Ryman, a highly respected aromatherapist with whom I had the priviledge of working with many years
ago, for kindling a fascination with the healing powers of plants and flowers.

To Peter Conway Grim, director of the College of Phytotherapy, London, and to Katherine Kong Jackson (Chinese
Herbal Medicine) far being so generous with their specialist knowledge.